Contents

HONEY WHEAT BREAD 9
GOOD WHITE BREAD 10
SHREDDED WHEAT BREAD 11
TUSCAN BREAD 12
RYE BREAD WITH ONION AND CARAWAY SEEDS 13
POTATO BREAD WITH ROSEMARY 15
OLIVE OIL AND BASIL BREAD 16
FOCACCIA WITH ROSEMARY 17
CHALLAH BREAD 18
COCONUT AND HAZELNUT BREAD 19
HONEY AND SESAME BAGELS 20
SWEET CORN BREAD 21
CINNAMON RAISIN BREAD 22
CRANBERRY WALNUT BREAD 23
DATE AND NUT BREAD 24
ZUCCHINI BREAD 24
ANDERSONS' FAMOUS BARBECUE SAUCE 25
ANDERSONS' FAMOUS STEAK SAUCE 26
TEXAS - STYLE BARBECUE SAUCE 26
SPICY BARBECUE SAUCE 27
FRESH CORN RELISH 27
FRESH TOMATO SALSA 28
SPICY AVOCADO DIP 29
HORSERADISH CREAM FOR STEAKS 29
ROASTED SHALLOT SALAD 29
BASIC PESTO 30
HUMMUS 30
ROASTED GARLIC HUMMUS 30

BABA GANOUJ	31
ORANGE GINGER MARINADE FOR CHICKEN	31
BALSAMIC VINEGAR AND MUSTARD MARINADE	32
PEANUT DIPPING SAUCE	32
ORANGE DIPPING SAUCE	33
BASIL MAYONNAISE	33
GARLIC MAYONNAISE	34
SUN-DRIED TOMATO MAYONNAISE	34
RASPBERRY MAYONNAISE	35
CRANBERRY CONSERVE	35
HOLIDAY CRANBERRY SAUCE	36
ALL-PURPOSE VEGETABLE STOCK	36
DOUBLE CHICKEN SOUP	37
TOMATO SOUP	38
ASPARAGUS SOUP	38
RED PEPPER SOUP	39
LEEK AND POTATO SOUP	39
SWEET CORN CHOWDER	40
MUSHROOM SOUP	41
CREAM OF MUSHROOM SOUP	41
SQUASH AND APPLE SOUP	42
LENTIL SOUP	43
TUSCAN BEAN SOUP	43
PASTA E FAGIOLI	44
MINESTRONE	45
COLD CUCUMBER SOUP	46
MELON SOUP WITH CALVADOS	46
MELON AND RASPBERRY SOUP	46
COLE SLAW WITH FRESH HORSERADISH	47
ASPARAGUS SALAD	47

TABBOULEH	48
COUSCOUS SALAD	49
CUCUMBER SALAD WITH TAHINI DRESSING	49
PICKLED CUCUMBER SALAD	50
ORZO AND SHRIMP SALAD	50
SALADE NIÇOISE	51
SHRIMP SALAD WITH AVOCADO AND GRAPEFRUIT	52
HEALTHY TUNA SALAD	52
CLASSIC TUNA SALAD	53
RED POTATO SALAD WITH SWEET ONIONS	53
WARM NEW POTATO AND SHIITAKE MUSHROOM SALAD	54
GREEN BEAN AND SWEET POTATO SALAD	54
POTATO AND EGG SALAD	55
HEALTHY POTATO SALAD	55
CLASSIC EGG SALAD	56
CHICKEN SALAD IN RADICCHIO LEAVES	56
CHICKEN SALAD WITH MANGO DRESSING	57
CLASSIC CHICKEN SALAD	58
AVOCADO AND BEAN SALAD	58
BLACK BEAN SALAD	58
LENTIL SALAD	59
TUSCAN BEAN SALAD	59
BROILED SEA BASS	60
STRIPED BASS WITH BRAISED TOMATO	60
BAKED WHOLE RED SNAPPER OR SEA BASS	61
CAJUN SWORDFISH STEAKS	62
BAKED FLOUNDER WITH FENNEL SAUCE	62
FLOUNDER POACHED IN TOMATO AND WINE	63
FLOUNDER BAKED IN PARCHMENT	64
OVEN-ROASTED SALMON WITH TOMATOES AND ASPARAGUS	64

SALMON IN A BASIL BUTTER SAUCE	65
GRILLED SALMON STEAKS WITH HERBED BUTTER	65
COLD POACHED SALMON WITH CUCUMBER DILL SAUCE	66
SALMON CAKES	67
SEARED SCALLOPS WITH SPRING VEGETABLES	67
MUSHROOM, TOMATO, AND SHRIMP OMELET	68
CHICKEN WITH MUSTARD SAUCE	69
BALSAMIC GLAZED CHICKEN	69
WHITE WINE BRAISED CHICKEN	70
BORDEAUX BRAISED CHICKEN	70
BAKED CHICKEN WITH APPLE CIDER AND APPLES	71
CHICKEN BREASTS STUFFED WITH WILD MUSHROOMS	72
CHICKEN TENDERS	73
GRILLED LEMON CHICKEN	73
CHICKEN BREASTS IN A PEANUT SAUCE	74
BROILED CHICKEN WITH MUSTARD AND HORSERADISH	74
TANDOORI-STYLE CHICKEN	75
ROASTED PEPPERS STUFFED WITH CHICKEN	75
CHICKEN SCALOPPINE WITH MUSHROOMS	76
TWO CHICKEN STEW	77
CHICKEN CURRY WITH COCONUT MILK	78
HUNTER'S CHICKEN	79
BULGUR STUFFING	79
CHESTNUT STUFFING	80
JALAPEÑO CORNBREAD STUFFING	81
TURKEY BREAST WITH CORNBREAD STUFFING	82
POT ROAST	83
BEEF STROGANOFF WITH NOODLES	84
FLANK STEAK WITH PORTOBELLO MUSHROOMS AND WINE	85
MARINATED PORK TENDERLOIN	85

- SPICY PORK TENDERLOIN ... 86
- PORK TENDERLOIN WITH MUSHROOM AND HERB SAUCE ... 87
- PORK VINDALOO ... 88
- TUSCAN-STYLE BRAISED PORK LOIN ... 89
- GREEN CHILI STEW ... 89
- BRAISED PORK CHOPS WITH PORTOBELLO MUSHROOMS ... 90
- PORK CHOPS WITH TOMATOES AND PEPPERS ... 90
- PORK CHOPS WITH APPLES ... 91
- STUFFED PORK CHOPS ... 92
- MELISSA FLOOD' S PULLED PORK ... 93
- RIB S ... 94
- VEAL CHOPS WITH MUSHROOMS AND PARSLEY ... 94
- VEAL CHOPS WITH RED PEPPER SAUCE ... 95
- VEAL CHOPS WITH SOUR CHERRY AND PORT WINE SAUCE ... 96
- BRAISED DOUBLE THICK VEAL CHOPS ... 96
- ROASTED VEAL WITH SHALLOTS ... 97
- BRAISED VEAL LOIN WITH SAGE AND PEARS ... 98
- OSSO BUCO ... 98
- VEAL SCALOPPINE ... 99
- IRISH LAMB STEW ... 100
- SHISH KEBABS ... 101
- MEATBALLS ... 102
- GREEN PEPPERS STUFFED WITH MEAT AND RICE ... 102
- MEATLOAF ... 103
- SOUTHWEST-STYLE RICE ... 104
- SHEPHERD'S PIE ... 104
- MOUSSAKA ... 105
- VEALBURGERS ... 107
- CHILI CON CARNE ... 107
- TARRAGON ROASTED VEGETABLES ... 108

RATATOUILLE	109
EGGPLANT AND PEPPERS	109
FRESH MOZZARELLA AND TOMATO NAPOLEON	110
VEGETARIAN TERRINE	110
REFRIED BLACK BEANS	111
FRIED GREEN TOMATOES	112
SAUTÉED MUSHROOMS	112
ASPARAGUS WITH LEMON BROTH	113
SPAGHETTI SQUASH WITH VEGETABLE MARINARA	113
VEGETARIAN VINDALOO	114
STUFFED ACORN SQUASH	115
ITALIAN ZUCCHINI	116
POTATO PANCAKES	117
HOT PEPPER PANCAKES	118
SCALLION PANCAKES	118
MUSHROOM PANCAKES	119
FRITTATA	120
ASPARAGUS FRITTATA	120
HORSERADISH MASHED POTATOES	121
BASIL MASHED POTATOES	122
WHIPPED POTATOES WITH ROSEMARY AND ROASTED GARLIC	122
POTATOES ROSTI	123
SWEET POTATO SUPREME	124
SWEET POTATOES, CARROTS, AND SQUASH	124
CHESTNUT CREAM	125
ONION TART	125
MUSHROOM AND ONION QUICHE	126
BRUSCHETTA	127
EGG NOODLES WITH PEAS AND GARLIC DRESSING	128
ASPARAGUS AND SPINACH WITH PASTA	128

SHRIMP WITH PASTA AND PESTO	129
CHICKEN AND PASTA SALAD WITH VEGETABLES	129
STUFFED SHELLS WITH SPINACH AND PARSLEY	130
CHICKEN AND SUN-DRIED TOMATOES WITH PASTA	132
RISOTT O	132
BASIL RISOTTO	133
ROASTED TOMATO RISOTTO	133
CARAMELIZED ONION RISOTTO	134
RISOTTO WITH ACORN SQUASH, SAGE, AND CHICKEN	135
LENTILS, RICE, AND ONIONS	135
ORZO WITH SUMMER VEGETABLES	136
BASIC TOMATO SAUCE	137
MEAT SAUCE FOR PASTA	137
FRESH TOMATO SAUCE	138
GRILLED PEPPER AND TOMATO SAUCE	138
PASTA SAUCE WITH SUN-DRIED TOMATOES	139
FESTIVE TOMATO SAUCE	140
PIZZA DOUGH	140
BASIC PIZZA	141
SPRING AND SUMMER PIZZA	142
FRESH PIZZA	143
BERRY PIE	144
AMARETTO CREAM PIE	144
LEMON CUPS	145
BOURBON BREAD PUDDING	146
RICE PUDDING	146
AMARETTO APPLE CRISP	147
BLUEBERRY COBBLER	148
APPLE WALNUT CAKE	148
ANGEL FOOD CAKE	149

PINEAPPLE UPSIDE-DOWN CAKE	150
GINGERBREAD	151
FRUIT SALAD WITH PORT	152
PEARS IN WINE	152
POACHED PEACHES	153
DRUNKEN BANANAS	153
MAPLE WALNUT BAKED APPLES	153
LIGHT LEMON SAUCE	154
UNFORGETTABLE FUDGE SAUCE	154
GOOD MACAROONS	155
CURRANT COCONUT CASHEW COOKIES	155
LEMON COCONUT COOKIES	156
MOLASSES COOKIES	157
OUR FAVORITE OATMEAL COOKIE	157
PEANUT BUTTER COOKIES	158
AUNT LEN'S CHRISTMAS COOKIES	158
PECAN PUFFS	159
THE BEST BROWNIES	160
SNICKERDOODLES	160

HONEY WHEAT BREAD

INGREDIENTS

- 2 packages (4 1/2 tsp.) dry yeast
- 2 c. lukewarm water
- 1/4 c. vegetable oil
- 1/4 c. honey
- 1 c. whole-wheat flour
- 1/2 c. cornmeal
- 2 tsp. vital wheat gluten (optional)
- 2 1/2 to 3 c. white bread flour

DIRECTIONS:

1. Dissolve the yeast in 1/2 cup of lukewarm water. When it begins to foam, add the rest of the water, oil, and honey, and stir to blend. In a separate bowl, combine the whole-wheat flour, cornmeal, and vital wheat gluten. Add them to the liquid mixture, stirring to combine. Then begin adding the white bread flour, 1/2 cup at a time, to create a stiff dough. When it becomes too hard to handle in the bowl, turn it out onto a floured surface and knead for 10 minutes or more, adding small amounts of white bread flour to prevent sticking, to create a smooth, elastic dough. (Or you can use an electric mixer with a dough hook. Pour in the liquid ingredients; add the whole-wheat flour, cornmeal, and vital wheat gluten and mix for a minute. Then add the white bread flour, 1/2 cup at a time, until the dough clings together and cleans the side of the bowl. Remove from the mixer bowl and knead a few times by hand to give the dough a uniform texture.) Lightly oil a straight-sided bowl, put the dough in it, cover it with plastic wrap, and put it in a warm place to rise until double in bulk. This should take about 1 hour.

2. When the dough has risen, punch it down, remove it from the bowl, knead it a few times, and return it to the bowl to rise for a second time, about 45 minutes.

3. When the dough has finished rising for the second time, turn it out of the bowl onto a floured surface. Divide it into two equal portions. Using your fingertips or the heel of your palm, flatten one piece of the dough into a large circle. Starting at the top of the circle, fold it toward you by quarters, pressing together the seam of each fold, to create a cylinder. Then fold the ends of the cylinder to the center, pressing together the seams, to create a loaf. Press the loaf into a lightly greased 4 1/2" × 9" loaf pan, seams side down. Repeat with the second piece of dough. Cover the loaf pans loosely with plastic wrap (sprinkle a little flour on top of each loaf to prevent the plastic wrap from sticking) and set them aside in a warm place to rise for the third time.

4. Preheat the oven to 450 degrees. When the loaves have doubled in bulk (about 1/2 hour), use a sharp knife to make three diagonal slashes across the top of each one. Then put them on the

bottom rack of the oven. Bake for 10 minutes at 450 degrees, then reduce the heat to 350 degrees and continue baking for another 25 to 30 minutes until the tops are well browned and the loaves sound hollow when thumped on the bottom, or a long toothpick or bamboo skewer inserted into the middle of a loaf comes out clean.

YIELD: 2 loaves
SODIUM CONTENT: less than 1 mg. of sodium per 1/2-inch slice

GOOD WHITE BREAD

INGREDIENTS
- 1 1/2 c. milk
- 1/2 c. semolina flour
- 2 packages (4 1/2 tsp.) dry yeast
- 1 1/2 c. water
- 2 tbsp. honey
- 2 tsp. vital wheat gluten (optional)
- 2 tbsp. unsalted butter, melted
- 4 c. white bread flour

DIRECTIONS:

1. Heat the milk in a small saucepan until almost boiling, then add the semolina flour and stir until the mixture thickens into a mush. Continue to stir so that there are no lumps, then set the pan aside to cool. Make sure it has cooled completely before adding to the dough.

2. Dissolve the yeast in 1/2 cup of lukewarm water and allow it to stand until foamy. Stir in the honey, add the rest of the water and the vital wheat gluten (if you are using it), then add the semolina mush, followed by the melted butter; stir to combine. Use a wooden spoon to stir in 2 to 3 cups of the flour. When the mixture gets too stiff to handle in the bowl, turn it out on a floured board and knead for several minutes, continuing to add small amounts of flour, until the dough becomes smooth and pliable. (Or use an electric mixer fitted with a dough hook to knead the dough. After the dough becomes too stiff to handle with a wooden spoon, transfer it to the mixer bowl, turn the mixer on to slow speed and add small amounts of additional flour until the ball of dough cleans the side of the bowl.) Transfer the dough to a lightly oiled straight-sided bowl, cover loosely with plastic wrap, and set aside to rise until more than double in bulk; this should take about an hour.

3. When the dough has risen, punch it down, remove it from the bowl, knead it a few times, and return it to the bowl to rise for a second time, about 45 minutes.

4. When the dough has finished rising for the second time, turn it out of the bowl onto a floured surface. Divide it into two equal portions. Using your fingertips or the heel of your palm, flatten one piece of the dough into a large circle. Starting at the top of the circle, fold it toward you by quarters, pressing together the seam of each fold, to create a cylinder. Then

fold the ends of the cylinder to the center, pressing together the seams, to create a loaf. Press the loaf into a lightly greased 41/2" × 9" loaf pan, seams side down. Repeat with the second piece of dough. Cover the loaf pans loosely with plastic wrap (sprinkle a little flour on top of each loaf to prevent the plastic wrap from sticking) and set them aside in a warm place to rise for the third time.

5. While they are rising, preheat the oven to 375 degrees. When the loaves have doubled in bulk (about 1/2 hour), use a sharp knife to cut three diagonal slashes in the top of each one, then put them on the bottom rack of the oven and bake until the tops are well browned—35 to 40 minutes. The bread is done when it sounds hollow if thumped on the bottom or a long toothpick or bamboo skewer inserted into the center of a loaf comes out clean.

YIELD : 2 loaves
SODIUM CONTENT: 7 mg. of sodium per 1/2-inch slice

SHREDDED WHEAT BREAD

INGREDIENTS
- 3 biscuits shredded wheat or 3 to 4 oz. bite-sized pieces
- 2 c. boiling water
- 2 tsp. vegetable oil
- 1/4 c. honey or molasses
- 2 packages (2 tbsp.) dry yeast
- 1/2 c. lukewarm water
- 5 to 6 c. all-purpose flour

DIRECTIONS:

1. Crumble up the shredded wheat in a large bowl, pour the boiling water over it, and stir to soften the fibers. Stir in the oil and the honey or molasses and set aside to cool. In a small bowl, dissolve the yeast in the lukewarm water. When the shredded wheat mixture has cooled completely, pour in the yeast mixture and stir to blend. Stir in the flour, 1/2 cup at a time, until the dough becomes too stiff to handle in the bowl. Turn it out on a floured board and knead for several minutes, continuing to add small amounts of flour, until the dough becomes smooth and pliable. (Or use an electric mixer fitted with a dough hook to knead the dough. After the dough becomes too stiff to handle with a wooden spoon, transfer it to the mixer bowl, turn the mixer on to slow speed and add small amounts of additional flour until the ball of dough cleans the side of the bowl.) Transfer the dough to a lightly oiled straight-sided bowl, cover loosely with plastic wrap, and set aside to rise until more than double in bulk; this should take about an hour.

2. When the dough has risen, punch it down, remove it from the bowl, knead it a few times, and return it to the bowl to rise for a second time, about 45 minutes.

3. When the dough has finished rising for the second time, turn it out of the bowl onto a floured

surface. Divide it into two equal portions. Using your fingertips or the heel of your palm, flatten one piece of the dough into a large circle. Starting at the top of the circle, fold it towards you by quarters, pressing together the seam of each fold, to create a cylinder. Then fold the ends of the cylinder to the center, pressing together the seams, to create a loaf. Press the loaf into a lightly greased 41/2" × 9" loaf pan, seams side down. Repeat with the second piece of dough. Cover the loaf pans loosely with plastic wrap (sprinkle a little flour on top of each loaf to prevent the plastic wrap from sticking), and set them aside in a warm place to rise for the third time.

4. While they are rising, preheat the oven to 375 degrees. When the loaves have doubled in bulk (about 1/2 hour), use a sharp knife to cut three diagonal slashes in the top of each one, then put them on the bottom rack of the oven and bake until the tops are well browned—35 to 40 minutes. The bread is done when it sounds hollow if thumped on the bottom or a long toothpick or bamboo skewer inserted into the center of a loaf comes out clean.

YIELD : 2 loaves
SODIUM CONTENT: 1 mg. of sodium per 1/2-inch slice

TUSCAN BREAD

INGREDIENTS

- 2 packages (41/2 tsp.) dry yeast
- 2 c. warm water
- 4 to 5 c. all-purpose flour
- 1 c. whole-wheat flour

DIRECTIONS:

1. Put the yeast and 1/2 cup of the warm water in a bowl and allow to stand for a few minutes, until the yeast dissolves. Then add the rest of the water and 1 cup of the white flour. Stir and allow to stand until foamy. Then add the whole-wheat flour and more white flour, handful by handful, until the mixture becomes too stiff to stir with a spoon.

2. Remove from the bowl and knead by hand, adding the rest of the flour in small amounts. This should take several minutes. Or put the dough in the bowl of an electric mixer and knead with a dough hook, adding small amounts of flour until the dough cleans the side of the bowl.

3. Lightly oil the sides of a clean bowl, put the kneaded dough in it, and cover it with plastic wrap. Put the dough in a warm place to rise. When it has doubled in bulk, remove from the bowl and knead for a few minutes. Then flatten it out on a floured surface so that it forms a large circle. Starting at the top of the circle, roll the dough toward you, using your hands to shape it into an oblong loaf. Press together the seams created by the folds of dough.

4. Spread flour on a dish towel and wrap it loosely around the loaf while it rises for the second time, until about doubled in size.

5. Place a baking tile on the bottom rack of the oven and preheat the oven to 400 degrees. When the dough has risen for the second time, open the oven door and quickly roll the dough out of the towel and onto the baking tile. (If you don't have a baking tile, you can bake the bread on a baking sheet lined with baker's parchment or sprinkled with a mixture of flour and cornmeal. Preheat the oven, roll the loaf out of the towel and onto the baking sheet on your kitchen counter, then put the baking sheet on the bottom rack of the oven.) When the loaf is in the oven, toss three or four ice cubes onto the oven floor and close the door. Don't open the door to peek at the bread for at least 20 minutes. Bake the bread for about 45 minutes or until it sounds hollow if thumped on the bottom or a long toothpick or bamboo skewer inserted into the center of a loaf comes out clean.
6. Allow the loaf to cool completely before cutting. The crust may soften as the bread cools. If you want a crisper crust, return the bread to the oven for a few minutes.

YIELD: 1 large loaf
SODIUM CONTENT: 2 mg. of sodium per 1/2-inch slice

RYE BREAD WITH ONION AND CARAWAY SEEDS

INGREDIENTS
FOR THE SPONGE:
- 2 packages (4 1/2 tsp.) dry yeast
- 1 1/2 c. lukewarm water
- 1 c. rye flour
- 1 c. bread flour
- 1 tbsp. caraway seeds
- 1/2 c. chopped onion

FOR THE DOUGH:
- all of the sponge
- 1 1/2 c. lukewarm water
- 2 tbsp. vegetable oil
- 2 tbsp. molasses
- 1 tbsp. caraway seeds
- 1 c. rye flour
- 4 to 5 c. bread flour

DIRECTIONS:
1. To prepare the sponge, dissolve the yeast in 1/2 cup of the lukewarm water in a large bowl; allow to sit for a few minutes until it begins to foam. Mix together the rye flour, bread flour,

and caraway seeds in a separate bowl. Add the rest of the water to the yeast mixture and stir to combine. Then add the flour mixture, 1/2 cup at a time, stirring until thoroughly blended. Bundle the onion in a piece of cheesecloth and tie at the top so that the onion pieces can't escape into the sponge. Push the bundle of onion into the middle of the sponge so that it is completely immersed.

2. Cover the bowl loosely with plastic wrap and set aside at room temperature so that the sponge can develop flavor as it rises and falls. It may be used after 6 hours but will be fine if left overnight.

3. To make the dough, remove the onion bundle, scrape off any of the sponge that clings to it, and discard the bundle. Add 1 1/2 cups of water to the sponge and stir to combine. Then stir in the vegetable oil, molasses, and caraway seeds. Mix the rye and bread flours together in a separate bowl, then add them to the sponge mixture, 1/2 cup at a time, until the dough becomes too stiff to handle in the bowl. Remove and knead by hand (or in the bowl of an electric mixer fitted with a dough hook), adding more flour as necessary until the ingredients are well mixed and form a pliable dough. This should take about 10 minutes if kneading by hand; about 5 minutes, or until the dough cleans the sides of the bowl, with the electric mixer. Lightly oil the mixing bowl and return the dough to it. Cover loosely with plastic wrap and put it in a warm place to rise until doubled in bulk. This should take about 1 1/2 hours.

4. Punch down the risen dough in the bowl and turn it out onto a floured board. Knead it a few times and divide it into two equal portions. Using your fingertips or the heel of your palm, flatten one piece of the dough into a large circle. Starting at the top of the circle, fold it toward you by quarters, pressing together the seam of each fold, to create an oblong loaf. Push the ends in and seal the edges. Repeat with the second piece of dough. Line a heavy baking sheet with baker's parchment or sprinkle it with a mixture of flour and cornmeal, place the loaves on it, seams side down, and cover loosely with plastic wrap (sprinkle a little flour on top of each loaf to prevent the plastic wrap from sticking). Allow to rise until the loaves have nearly doubled in bulk, about 1/2 hour.

5. While the loaves are rising, place a baking tile (if you have one) on the bottom rack of the oven and preheat the oven to 425 degrees. When the loaves have risen, use a sharp knife or razor blade to cut three slashes about 1/2 inch deep diagonally across the top of each loaf. Put the baking sheet in the oven on the tile (or on the bottom rack if you aren't using a tile), toss two ice cubes on the floor of the oven, close the door, and do not open it to peek at the bread for at least 20 minutes. Allow the bread to bake for 35 to 40 minutes; it is done when it sounds hollow if thumped on the bottom or a long toothpick or bamboo skewer inserted into the center of a loaf comes out clean.

6. Allow the loaves to cool completely before cutting. The crust may soften as the bread cools. If you want a crisper crust, return the bread to the oven for a few minutes.

YIELD: 2 loaves

SODIUM CONTENT: 2 mg. of sodium per 1/2-inch slice

POTATO BREAD WITH ROSEMARY

- **Ingredients**
- 1 1/2 lbs. Yukon Gold or other full-flavored potatoes
- 2 packages (4 1/2 tsp.) dry yeast
- 1/4 c. warm water
- 3 to 4 c. all-purpose flour
- 2 tbsp. olive oil
- 1 heaping tbsp. chopped fresh rosemary leaves

DIRECTIONS:

1. Boil the potatoes in their skins until fork-tender. Then peel and mash or put through a ricer. Set aside to cool.

2. Prepare a sponge by dissolving the yeast in the warm water and adding 1 cup of the flour. (Add a tablespoon or two of water if the mixture seems too stiff.) Stir, cover with plastic wrap, and set aside in a warm place to rise until double in bulk (1 to 2 hours).

3. Stir down the sponge and transfer it to a large mixing bowl or the bowl of an electric mixer. Add the olive oil, potatoes, and rosemary, and stir to blend. Stir in the rest of the flour, a handful at a time, until the dough becomes too stiff to handle. Then transfer to a floured board and knead by hand, adding the rest of the flour in small amounts. Or knead with the mixer, using a dough hook, adding small amounts of flour until the dough cleans the sides of the bowl.

4. Lightly oil a clean bowl, put the kneaded dough in it, and cover with plastic wrap. Allow it to rise in a warm place until it has doubled in bulk. This should take about an hour. Punch down the dough, remove it from the bowl, and knead it for a few minutes. Divide into two equal portions. Use your fingertips or the heel of your palm to flatten one piece of dough into a circle. Fold the edges of the circle under it toward its center, rotating the dough with your hands, to form a high circular loaf. Repeat with the second piece of dough.

5. Line a heavy baking sheet with baker's parchment or sprinkle it with a mixture of flour and cornmeal, place the loaves on it, seam side down, and cover loosely with plastic wrap. (Sprinkle a little flour on top of the loaf to prevent the plastic wrap from sticking.) Allow to rise until nearly doubled in bulk, about a 1/2 hour.

6. While the loaves are rising, place a baking tile (if you have one) on the bottom rack of the oven and preheat the oven to 400 degrees. When the loaves have risen, use a sharp knife or razor blade to cut two slashes about 1/2 inch deep across the top of each one. Put the baking sheet in the oven on the tile (or on the bottom rack if you aren't using a tile). Bake for 35 to 40 minutes; the bread is done when it sounds hollow if thumped on the bottom or a long toothpick or bamboo skewer inserted into the center of the loaf comes out clean.

7. Allow the loaves to cool completely before cutting. The crust may soften as the bread cools.

If you want a crisper crust, return the bread to the oven for a few minutes.

YIELD: 2 loaves

SODIUM CONTENT: 3 mg. of sodium per 1/2-inch slice

OLIVE OIL AND BASIL BREAD

INGREDIENTS

- 2 tbsp. dry yeast
- 2 c. lukewarm water
- 1/2 c. good quality olive oil
- 1/4 c. chopped basil leaves
- 4 to 5 c. bread flour
- 1 tbsp. vital wheat gluten (optional)
- cornmeal

DIRECTIONS:

1. Dissolve the yeast in 1/2 cup of the lukewarm water and allow to stand until it begins to foam. Add the oil, basil leaves, and the rest of the water; stir. Add 2 cups of the flour and stir to blend until the mixture becomes too stiff to handle in the bowl. Remove and knead by hand (or in the bowl of an electric mixer fitted with a dough hook), adding more flour as necessary until the ingredients are well mixed and form a pliable dough. This should take about 10 minutes if kneading by hand, or about 5 minutes with the electric mixer, until the dough cleans the sides of the bowl. Lightly oil the mixing bowl and return the dough to it. Cover loosely with plastic wrap and put it in a warm place to rise until doubled in bulk. This should take about an hour.

2. When the dough has risen, punch it down, remove it from the bowl, and divide it into five equal sections. Using your fingertips, flatten each section into a circle. To form a small round loaf, fold the edges of the circle into the center, pinching the seams together. Then turn the loaf over on the board and rotate it between your palms to make the loaf rounder and higher. Pinch the seams on the bottom together before placing each loaf, seam side down, on a heavy baking sheet dusted with a mixture of flour and cornmeal. Spread a sheet of plastic wrap loosely over the loaves and let them rise again until double in bulk. (Sprinkle a bit of flour on top of each loaf to prevent the plastic wrap from sticking.) This should take about a 1/2 hour.

3. Place a baking tile (if you have one) on the bottom rack of the oven and preheat the oven to 375 degrees. When the loaves have risen, place the baking sheet on the tile (or on the bottom rack) and toss two ice cubes on the floor of the oven before closing the door. Bake for 30 minutes; the bread is done when it sounds hollow if thumped on the bottom or a long toothpick or bamboo skewer inserted into the center of a loaf comes out clean.

4. Allow the loaves to cool completely before cutting. The crust may soften as the bread cools. If you want a crisper crust, return the bread to the oven for a few minutes.

YIELD: 5 loaves of bread
SODIUM CONTENT: 2 mg. of sodium per slice

FOCACCIA WITH ROSEMARY

INGREDIENTS

- 3 packages (6 3/4 tsps.) dry yeast
- 2 c. lukewarm water
- 4 c. all-purpose flour
- 1/3 c. plus 2 tbsp. olive oil
- 1 tbsp. finely chopped fresh rosemary
- 1 tbsp. whole rosemary leaves

DIRECTIONS:

1. Dissolve the yeast in 1 cup of the lukewarm water. Add 1 cup of the flour and stir to blend into a paste. Cover this "sponge" and set it aside in a warm area until double in bulk; this should take about an hour.

2. Put the sponge in a large mixing bowl, add the rest of the water, and stir to blend. Then add 1/3 cup of the oil and the chopped rosemary. Add more of the flour until the dough becomes too stiff to handle in the bowl. Turn it out on a floured board and knead in the rest of the flour. Continue kneading for a few more minutes until the dough achieves a uniform, elastic texture. (Or put the dough in the bowl of an electric mixer fitted with a dough hook and use it to knead in the rest of the flour until the dough cleans the sides of the bowl.) Put the dough in a lightly oiled bowl, cover loosely with plastic wrap, and set aside in a warm place to rise until double in bulk; this should take about 1 1/2 hours.

3. You can cook all the dough on a rectangular 15" × 11" jellyroll pan or you can divide it into two pieces and cook them in straight-sided 9-inch cake tins that have been brushed lightly with olive oil. Punch down the dough and, if dividing it, form it into two balls of equal size. Use a rolling pin to roll each ball into a circle about the diameter of the cake tin. Put the dough in the two tins and use your fingertips to spread the dough so that it reaches the sides of the tins. (If using a jellyroll pan, brush it lightly with olive oil, roll the dough into a large rectangle, put it in the pan, and spread it to reach the sides). Cover loosely with plastic wrap and set aside in a warm area to rise again until double in bulk. This should take 30 to 45 minutes.

4. While the dough is rising, preheat the oven to 350 degrees. When the dough has risen, sprinkle with the remaining 2 tablespoons of olive oil and "dimple" the surface, spreading your fingers and pushing down firmly with them until they touch the bottom of the pan. Repeat to create an even pattern of holes in the dough separated from each other by an inch. Sprinkle with the whole rosemary leaves. Put the focaccia in the oven and bake for about 20 minutes, or until the crust turns golden brown.

YIELD : 10 slices
SODIUM CONTENT: 10 mg. of sodium per slice

CHALLAH BREAD

INGREDIENTS

- 2 packages (4 1/2 tsp.) dry yeast
- 2 c. lukewarm water
- 3 eggs
- 2 tbsp. sugar
- 2 tbsp. honey
- 3 tbsp. unsalted butter, melted
- 5 to 6 c. bread flour
- 1 tbsp. milk
- poppy seeds

DIRECTIONS:

1. Dissolve the yeast in 1/2 cup of the lukewarm water and allow to stand until it begins to foam. Break two of the eggs into another bowl and beat them lightly. Add the rest of the water, sugar, honey, and melted butter. (Make sure the butter has cooled and add it slowly so that it doesn't cook the eggs.) When the yeast mixture has turned frothy, stir it into the rest of the ingredients. Stir in the flour, 1/2 cup at a time, until the dough gets too stiff to stir in the bowl.

2. Turn the dough out on a floured board and knead in the rest of the flour so that the dough becomes smooth and elastic. Continue to knead for another 5 minutes. (Or, if you prefer, stir 2 cups of flour into the wet ingredients, put the mixture into the bowl of an electric mixer fitted with a dough hook, and use it to mix and knead in the rest of the flour, adding 1/2 cup at a time until the dough cleans the sides of the bowl.) Put the dough into a lightly oiled bowl, cover loosely with plastic wrap, and set aside in a warm place to rise until doubled in bulk. This should take 1 to 1 1/2 hours.

3. Divide the dough in half, then divide each half into three pieces. Roll each piece of dough into a ball. Take a ball of dough, flatten it on a floured board, and roll it into a cylinder. Then continue to roll the cylinder, pushing out from the middle toward the ends, to form a round strip of dough about a foot long. Repeat with two more balls of dough. When you have three foot-long strips of dough, line them up side by side and pinch one set of ends together. Then braid the dough strips together, as if braiding rope or hair, and pinch the other ends together. Fold the ends under the braided loaf and place it in a lightly greased loaf pan. Repeat with the other three balls of dough.

4. Break the third egg into a bowl, add the milk, and beat to combine. Use a pastry brush to daub the egg mixture on top of each loaf. Sprinkle the loaves with poppy seeds, drape a piece

of plastic wrap loosely over them, and set them aside to rise for about 1/2 hour, until doubled in bulk.

5. Preheat the oven to 400 degrees. Put the loaves on the bottom rack of the oven and bake for 30 to 40 minutes, until the tops have turned a rich golden brown and a thump on the bottom of a loaf produces a hollow sound or a long toothpick or bamboo skewer inserted into the middle of a loaf comes out clean.

YIELD : 2 loaves

SODIUM CONTENT: 10 mg. of sodium per 1/2-inch slice

COCONUT AND HAZELNUT BREAD

INGREDIENTS

- 3/4 c. shredded coconut
- 2 packages (4 1/2 tsp.) dry yeast
- 3/4 c. lukewarm water
- 1/4 c. honey
- 2 eggs
- 4 tbsp. (1/2 stick) unsalted butter
- 3 c. bread flour
- 3/4 c. chopped hazelnuts
- 1 egg white

DIRECTIONS:

1. Preheat the oven to 350 degrees. Spread the coconut in a baking pan and toast in the oven for about 5 minutes or until it begins to turn golden brown, then remove and allow to cool. Dissolve the yeast in 1/2 cup of the water and allow to stand until it begins to foam. Then add the rest of the water, the honey, the eggs, and the butter; stir until well blended. Add 2 cups of the flour, 1/2 cup at a time, stirring to blend. Then stir in all but 1 tablespoon of the coconut and all but 1 tablespoon of the chopped hazelnuts.

2. Add the remaining flour in small amounts until the dough becomes too stiff to handle in the bowl. Then turn it out onto a floured board and knead by hand for several minutes, adding flour, until it holds together and feels elastic. (Or transfer the dough to the bowl of a mixer fitted with a dough hook and knead at slow speed, adding small amounts of flour, until the dough cleans the sides of the bowl.) After it is kneaded, put the dough in a lightly greased, straight-sided bowl, cover loosely with plastic wrap, and set aside to rise until double in bulk, about an hour.

3. When the dough has risen, punch it down, remove it from the bowl, and use your fingertips and the heel of your palm to flatten it so that it forms a large oval. Fold it toward you from the top to form a cylinder, pinching together the seam along the bottom. Then turn it seam side up and fold the ends to the center, pinching together the seams again, to form a loaf. Put

the loaf seam-side down in an 8" × 4" loaf pan and press down the top of the loaf so that it fills out the pan. Sprinkle flour lightly on top of the loaf, cover loosely with plastic wrap, and set aside to rise for the second time until double in bulk, about 1/2 an hour.

4. While the loaf is rising, preheat the oven to 350 degrees. When the loaf has risen, use a sharp knife to cut a single slash about 1/2 inch deep down the center of it lengthwise. Mix the egg white with a little water and brush the top of the loaf lightly with the mixture. Then sprinkle the top with the reserved coconut and hazelnuts. Bake on the bottom rack of the oven for 30 to 40 minutes, until the top is golden brown and the loaf sounds hollow when thumped on the bottom or a bamboo skewer inserted into the center of the loaf comes out clean.

5. Allow the loaf to cool completely before cutting. The crust may soften as the bread cools. If you want a crisper crust, return the bread to the oven for a few minutes.

YIELD : 1 large loaf

SODIUM CONTENT: 15 mg. of sodium per 1/2-inch slice

HONEY AND SESAME BAGELS

INGREDIENTS

FOR THE SPONGE:

- 2 packages (4 1/2 tsp.) dry yeast
- 2 c. lukewarm water
- 2 c. all-purpose flour

FOR THE BAGELS:

- 2 tbsp. vegetable oil
- 2 tbsp. honey
- 1 1/2 c. water
- 1/2 c. semolina flour
- 3 to 4 c. all-purpose flour
- 1 gallon water
- sesame seeds

DIRECTIONS:

1. Prepare a sponge by dissolving the yeast in 1/2 cup of the lukewarm water, allowing it to stand for a few minutes until it begins to foam. Then add the remaining 1 1/2 cups of lukewarm water, stir, and add 2 cups of all-purpose flour. Stir for 100 strokes, until well blended. Cover with plastic wrap and set aside in a warm place for about 2 hours. During this time, it should rise and fall and acquire a bubbly texture.

2. Mix the vegetable oil and honey with 1 1/2 cups of water. When the sponge is ready, add this mixture to it and stir to blend thoroughly. Stir in the semolina flour, then add the all-purpose flour, 1/2 cup at a time, stirring to blend until the mixture becomes too stiff to handle. Turn it

out onto a floured board and knead for several minutes, adding more flour in small amounts until the dough is smooth and elastic. (Or transfer the mixture to the bowl of an electric mixer after adding the semolina, insert the dough hook and use the mixer to knead in the all-purpose flour, adding it by the 1/2 cup until the ball of dough cleans the sides of the bowl.)

3. Lightly oil the sides of a straight-sided bowl, put the dough in it, cover loosely with plastic wrap, and put in a warm place to rise until double in bulk. This should take 1 1/2 to 2 hours. Check the dough to see how fast it is rising, and about 20 minutes before it has completed its rise, put the gallon of water in a large pot over high heat so that it will boil by the time the dough has risen. Lightly grease two baking sheets and preheat the oven to 375 degrees.

4. When the dough has risen, punch it down, remove it from the bowl, and divide it into two equal parts. Then divide each part into eight equal portions. Roll each small piece of dough between your palms to form a cylinder several inches long, then form it into a circle by pinching the ends together. When you have shaped four bagels in this way, drop them, one by one, into the boiling water. They should sink to the bottom for a few seconds, then rise to the top. Allow them to remain in the simmering water for about a minute before using a slotted spoon or spatula to remove them to one of the baking sheets. Repeat the process for the rest of the dough pieces, four at a time.

5. Put eight bagels on each baking sheet. Sprinkle them generously with sesame seeds. Put them on the bottom rack of the oven and cook for about 30 minutes, or until they have turned a rich golden brown.

YIELD : 16 bagels
SODIUM CONTENT: 3 mg. of sodium per bagel

SWEET CORN BREAD

- **Ingredients**
- 1 egg
- 1/2 c. plain yogurt
- 1/2 c. milk
- 3 tbsp. melted butter
- 3 tbsp. honey
- 1 c. fresh corn (or frozen unsalted corn)
- 1 c. yellow or blue cornmeal
- 1 c. all-purpose flour
- 4 tsp. low-sodium baking powder

DIRECTIONS:

1. Preheat the oven to 350 degrees. Grease an 8-inch square baking pan. Stir together the egg, yogurt, milk, butter, honey, and corn in a large bowl until well blended. Sift together the

cornmeal, flour, and baking powder in a separate bowl and add them to the mixture of wet ingredients. Stir only until the dry ingredients are moistened. Pour the batter into the pan and bake for 20 to 25 minutes, until a toothpick inserted into the center of the cornbread comes out clean.

YIELD : 12 pieces
SODIUM CONTENT: 19 mg. of sodium per piece

CINNAMON RAISIN BREAD

- **Ingredients**
- 2 packages (4 1/2 tsp.) dry yeast
- 2 1/4 c. lukewarm water
- 1 c. raisins
- 1 c. whole-wheat flour
- 3 c. white flour
- 1/3 c. honey
- 1/4 c. vegetable oil
- 1/4 c. cinnamon
- 1/4 c. sugar
- 2 tbsp. melted butter

DIRECTIONS:

1. Dissolve the yeast in 1/2 cup of the lukewarm water and let stand until it begins to foam. Combine the whole-wheat flour with 1 cup of the white flour in a large bowl. Add the raisins and stir to distribute them evenly through the flour. Stir the honey, oil, and the rest of the warm water into the yeast mixture, then pour it over the flour. Stir until blended. Add the rest of the white flour, 1/2 cup at a time, until the dough gets too stiff to handle in the bowl. Turn the dough out onto a floured board and knead for about 10 minutes, adding small amounts of flour, until it becomes smooth and elastic. (Or put the dough in the bowl of an electric mixer and knead with the dough hook, adding small amounts of flour, until it cleans the sides of the bowl.)

2. Lightly oil a clean bowl and put the dough in it, cover loosely with plastic wrap, and put it in a warm place to rise until the dough doubles in bulk, about 1 to 1 1/2 hours.

3. Punch down the dough and divide into two equal pieces. Flatten out the first piece on a floured board to make a large rectangle. Mix together the cinnamon and sugar and reserve 2 tablespoons to sprinkle on the finished loaves. Spread half of the rest generously over the flattened dough. Fold two ends of the dough over the center, as if folding a sheet of paper. Then roll up one end of the folded dough to make a cylinder. Pinch the ends of the cylinder together to form a loaf and place it, seam side down, in a lightly greased loaf pan. Repeat for

the second piece of dough. Cover the loaves loosely with plastic wrap (sprinkle a little flour on top of each one to prevent the plastic wrap from sticking). Put the loaves in a warm place to rise until almost double in size, about a 1/2 hour.

4. Preheat the oven to 325 degrees while the bread is rising. When it has risen, gently brush or blow the flour off the top of the loaves and brush them with melted butter. Then sprinkle them with the reserved sugar and cinnamon. Bake for about 30 minutes, or until the loaves sound hollow when tapped on the bottom or a long toothpick or bamboo skewer inserted into the middle of a loaf comes out clean.

YIELD : 2 loaves
  SODIUM CONTENT: 2 mg. of sodium per 1/2-inch slice

CRANBERRY WALNUT BREAD

- **Ingredients**
- 1 package (2 1/4 tsp.) dry yeast
- 1 c. lukewarm water
- 1/4 c. molasses
- 2 tbsp. honey
- 3/4 c. coarsely chopped walnuts
- 3/4 c. halved cranberries
- 3 tbsp. unsalted butter, melted
- 1/2 c. whole-wheat flour
- 2 to 3 c. white bread flour
- 1 tbsp. vital wheat gluten (optional)
- **DIRECTIONS**

1. Dissolve the yeast in 1/2 cup of the lukewarm water and let stand until it begins to foam. Add the rest of the water, the molasses, honey, walnuts, and cranberries and stir to blend. Stir in the whole-wheat flour and wheat gluten (if you are using it), then slowly add the melted butter, stirring constantly. Stir in the white flour, 1/2 cup at a time.

2. When the dough gets too stiff to handle in the bowl, turn it out onto a floured board and knead it by hand for several minutes, adding small amounts of flour, until it is smooth and elastic. (Or transfer the dough to the bowl of an electric mixer fitted with a dough hook and mix, adding small amounts of flour, until the dough cleans the sides of the bowl.) Put the kneaded dough in a lightly oiled straight-sided bowl and put it in a warm place to rise until double in bulk, about 1 to 1 1/2 hours.

3. Punch down the risen dough, knead it a few times, and divide it into two equal pieces. Using your fingertips or the heel of your palm, flatten a piece of the dough into a large oval. Starting at a narrow end, roll the dough up into a cylinder. Turn it seam side up, pinch the

ends tight and fold them into the center to form an oblong loaf. Place the loaf in a lightly greased loaf pan, seam side down. Dust the top of the loaf with flour, cover loosely with plastic wrap, and set aside to rise until double in bulk, about 20 to 30 minutes.

4. Preheat the oven to 450 degrees. When the loaf has risen, use a sharp knife to make a cut about 1/2 inch deep down the length of the top, then put the loaf on the bottom rack of the oven to bake. After 10 minutes, turn the oven temperature down to 350 degrees. Bake for another 30 minutes, until the loaf sounds hollow when thumped on the bottom or a long toothpick or bamboo skewer inserted into the loaf comes out clean.

YIELD : 1 loaf
SODIUM CONTENT: 4 mg. of sodium per 1/2-inch slice

DATE AND NUT BREAD

INGREDIENTS

- 3/4 c. chopped walnuts
- 1 c. chopped dates
- 1 tbsp. low-sodium baking powder
- 3 tbsp. vegetable shortening
- 3/4 c. boiling water
- 2 eggs
- 1 tsp. vanilla
- 1/2 c. white sugar
- 1/2 c. brown sugar
- 1 1/2 c. sifted all-purpose flour
- **DIRECTIONS**

1. Combine the walnuts, dates, and baking powder in a mixing bowl. Add the shortening and pour in the boiling water. Stir to distribute, then allow the mixture to stand for 20 minutes
2. .Preheat the oven to 350 degrees. Break the eggs into a large bowl and beat them briefly with a fork. Stir in the vanilla, sugars, and flour. Add the date-nut mixture, stirring to blend. Be sure the dates and nuts are distributed evenly through the batter. Grease a 9" × 5" loaf pan and pour the mixture into it. Bake for about 1 hour or until a toothpick inserted into the loaf comes out clean.

YIELD : 1 loaf
SODIUM CONTENT: 13 mg. of sodium per 1/2-inch slice

ZUCCHINI BREAD

INGREDIENTS

- 3 eggs

- 1 1/4 c. vegetable oil
- 1 1/2 c. sugar
- 1 tsp. vanilla
- 2 c. finely grated raw zucchini
- 2 c. all-purpose flour
- 3 1/2 tsp. low-sodium baking powder
- 1 tsp. ground cloves
- 1 tsp. ground cinnamon

DIRECTIONS:

1. Preheat the oven to 350 degrees. Combine the eggs, oil, sugar, and vanilla, and beat until well blended. Add zucchini and stir to combine. Sift the flour and baking powder together with the spices and stir into the oil mixture until the dry ingredients are moistened. Do not overmix. Spoon the batter into a lightly greased 9" × 5" loaf pan, taking care not to fill it more than three-quarters full. Put any leftover batter in a small greased baking dish. Cook for an hour or more on the middle rack of the oven until a toothpick dipped into the middle of the loaf comes out clean.

YIELD : 1 loaf
 SODIUM CONTENT: 19 mg. of sodium per 1/2-inch piece

IV. CONDIMENTS
ANDERSONS' FAMOUS BARBECUE SAUCE

INGREDIENTS
- 1 large onion, diced
- vegetable oil
- 28-oz. can salt-free tomato purée
- 2 fresh tomatoes, chopped
- 2 c. white wine vinegar
- 1/2 c. brown sugar
- freshly ground black pepper to taste
- 2 tbsp. paprika
- 2 tbsp. salt-free chili powder
- 1/4 c. molasses
- 1 c. pineapple juice

- 1/4 c. plus 2 tbsp. salt-free Dijon mustard
- 2 tbsp. dark rum
- 2 cloves garlic, minced

DIRECTIONS:

1. Sauté the onion in a little oil until translucent. Add the rest of the ingredients, stirring to blend well. Bring the mixture to a boil, then reduce the heat and simmer over very low heat for 3 to 4 hours.
2. Cool the sauce, then transfer it to a glass jar or bowl and refrigerate until ready to use.

YIELD : 8 cups of sauce
SODIUM CONTENT: 8 mg. of sodium per 1/4 cup

ANDERSONS' FAMOUS STEAK SAUCE

INGREDIENTS

- 8 medium tomatoes, quartered
- 1 tbsp. olive oil
- 1 shallot, minced
- 1/2 c. white wine vinegar
- 1/2 c. packed brown sugar
- 1/4 c. salt-free pickle relish
- 1/4 c. molasses
- 1/4 tsp. garlic powder
- **DIRECTIONS**

1. Place the quartered tomatoes in a blender and blend until liquefied. For a really smooth sauce, force the tomatoes through a fine strainer. Heat the oil in a pot to medium heat; add the shallot and cook for several minutes until wilted. Add the tomato and all the other ingredients to the pot; reduce to a simmer and cook for 2 1/2 to 3 hours.
2. Allow the sauce to cool, and refrigerate overnight before using.

YIELD : 6 cups of sauce
SODIUM CONTENT: 6 mg. of sodium per 1/4 cup

TEXAS - STYLE BARBECUE SAUCE

INGREDIENTS

- 2 tbsp. vegetable oil
- 1 onion, diced
- 1 c. salt-free catsup
- 28-oz. can salt-free tomatoes, chopped, or 3 large fresh tomatoes, chopped

- 1 c. white wine vinegar
- 1/4 c. molasses
- 1 tbsp. cayenne pepper
- 4 dried red chili peppers
- freshly ground black pepper to taste

DIRECTIONS:

1. Heat the oil in a large saucepan; add the onion and sauté over medium heat for 10 minutes. Then add the rest of the ingredients. Stir to combine. Simmer over low heat for at least an hour.

YIELD : 6 cups of sauce
SODIUM CONTENT: 13 mg. of sodium per 1/4 cup

SPICY BARBECUE SAUCE

INGREDIENTS

- 2 tbsp. oil
- 1 medium onion, chopped
- 4 jalapeño peppers, seeded and diced
- 1 tbsp. chopped fresh ginger
- 4 medium tomatoes, chopped
- 2 tbsp. honey
- 2 tbsp. white wine vinegar
- 1/2 tsp. dried coriander
- 1/2 tsp. dried cumin
- 1 c. fresh cilantro leaves

DIRECTIONS:

1. Heat the oil in a medium saucepan; add the onion, peppers, and ginger. Cook for 10 minutes over medium heat. Then add the rest of the ingredients and stir to combine. Bring the mixture to a simmer and cook for 45 minutes. If the vegetables don't release enough liquid to keep the mixture moist as it cooks, add a little water. Remove from the heat and let cool.
2. When cool, transfer the mixture to a blender or food processor and blend to a liquid. Brush the sauce onto meat before charcoal grilling or broiling in the oven, then use it to baste the meat as it is almost done. (Note: If you prefer a hotter sauce, add cayenne pepper to taste.)

YIELD : 3 cups of sauce
SODIUM CONTENT: 5 mg. of sodium per 1/4 cup

FRESH CORN RELISH

INGREDIENTS

- 4 ears fresh sweet corn, husked and silk removed, or 3 c. frozen salt-free corn
- 1 tbsp. olive oil
- 3 tbsp. diced red onion
- 2 tbsp. diced orange sweet pepper
- 2 tsp. balsamic vinegar
- freshly ground black pepper to taste

DIRECTIONS:

1. Strip the kernels from the corncobs by running a knife lengthwise down the ear of corn (or defrost the frozen corn). Heat the oil in a nonstick pan until moderately hot. Add the corn to the pan and cook, stirring frequently, for 2 minutes. Then add the rest of the ingredients and cook 1 minute longer. Remove from the heat and allow to cool before serving.

YIELD : About 1 3/4 cups
SODIUM CONTENT: 4 mg. of sodium per 1/4 cup

FRESH TOMATO SALSA

- **Ingredients**
- 6 ripe tomatoes
- 1/2 c. chopped red onion
- 1/4 c. chopped scallions
- 1 tbsp. finely minced garlic
- 1 tbsp. olive oil
- 1/4 c. chopped cilantro
- 2 tbsp. lime juice
- 1 tbsp. lemon juice
- 2 tbsp. cider vinegar
- 1 small jalapeño pepper, finely minced

DIRECTIONS:

1. Peel the tomatoes by dipping each one in a pot of boiling water for several seconds, then running it under cold water; this should loosen the skin so that it pulls off easily when pierced with a knife. Cut the tomatoes open, remove the seeds, and cut the flesh into pieces. Put the tomato, chopped onion, and chopped scallion in a blender or food processor and blend slowly or pulse to achieve a coarse blend. Pour the mixture into a bowl. Stir in the rest of the ingredients. Serve as an appetizer or snack with unsalted corn chips, or as a sauce for chicken or fish with rice.

YIELD : 4 cups

SODIUM CONTENT: 5 mg. of sodium per 1/4 cup

SPICY AVOCADO DIP

- **Ingredients**
- 3 ripe avocados, peeled
- juice of 1/2 lemon
- 2 jalapeño peppers, seeded and finely diced
- 1 shallot, finely diced

DIRECTIONS:

1. Slice the avocado into a bowl and mash it with a fork to create a lumpy paste. Add the lemon juice, jalapeño, and shallots; mix well to combine, and chill before serving.

YIELD : Serves 6

SODIUM CONTENT: 11 mg. of sodium per serving

HORSERADISH CREAM FOR STEAKS

INGREDIENTS

- 1/2 c. grated fresh horseradish root
- 1/3 c. sour cream
- freshly ground black pepper to taste
- 1 tbsp. lemon juice

DIRECTIONS:

1. Mix all the ingredients together and place in a serving dish.

YIELD : 1 cup

SODIUM CONTENT: 6 mg. of sodium per 2-tablespoon serving

ROASTED SHALLOT SALAD

- **Ingredients**
- 1 dozen shallots, ends removed, papery skin peeled off
- 2 tbsp. olive oil
- freshly ground black pepper to taste
- 3 tbsp. balsamic vinegar

DIRECTIONS:

1. Preheat the oven to 350 degrees. Put the shallots in an ovenproof baking dish, drizzle with oil, sprinkle with pepper, and bake for 1 hour and 15 minutes. Remove the pan from the oven; add the balsamic vinegar and stir to blend. Remove to a bowl; serve warm with meats.

YIELD : Serves 6

SODIUM CONTENT: 4 mg. of sodium per serving

BASIC PESTO

INGREDIENTS
- 2 c. chopped fresh basil
- 1/2 c. good quality olive oil
- 1/4 c. pine nuts or walnuts
- 2 cloves garlic

DIRECTIONS:
1. Blend all the ingredients in a food processor or blender until smooth. For a creamy texture, add a bit more oil.

HUMMUS

INGREDIENTS
- 2 c. chickpeas, cooked without salt, or 2 14-oz. cans unsalted chickpeas
- 2 cloves garlic, sliced
- 2/3 c. sesame tahini
- 2/3 c. lemon juice
- 1/4 c. olive oil
- 2 tbsp. chopped parsley

DIRECTIONS:
1. Blend all the ingredients except parsley in a blender or food processor to a smooth purée. Stir in the parsley or sprinkle it over the top before serving. Serve with triangles of toasted salt-free bread or salt-free pita pockets.

YIELD : 3 1/2 cups
SODIUM CONTENT: 9 mg. of sodium per 1/4 -cup serving

ROASTED GARLIC HUMMUS

- **Ingredients**
- 2 c. chickpeas cooked without salt or 2 (14-oz.) cans unsalted chickpeas
- 1 whole head of garlic
- 8 fresh basil leaves, chopped
- freshly ground black pepper to taste
- 1/4 c. low-sodium chicken broth
- juice of 1/2 lemon

DIRECTIONS:

1. Preheat the oven to 350 degrees. Put the head of garlic, whole, in a small baking dish and roast it until the cloves are soft; this should take about an hour. Remove the garlic from the oven and slice off the top, then squeeze the head over a small dish to extract the cooked garlic flesh from the papery skin. Combine the drained beans, cooked garlic, and the rest of the ingredients in a food processor and process to a smooth purée. Chill for an hour before serving.

YIELD : Serves 6
SODIUM CONTENT: 19 mg. of sodium per serving

BABA GANOUJ

INGREDIENTS
- 1 medium eggplant
- 3 cloves garlic, minced
- 1/4 c. sesame tahini
- 1/3 c. lemon juice
- freshly ground black pepper to taste
- sprigs of parsley for garnish

DIRECTIONS:
1. Preheat the oven to 350 degrees. Place the eggplant on a lightly greased baking sheet and put it in the oven to roast until the flesh inside it cooks through and it collapses on itself (about 45 minutes, depending on the size of the eggplant). After it has cooled, cut the eggplant open, scoop out the flesh and put it in a food processor or blender. Add the garlic, tahini, and lemon juice, and blend until smooth. Stir in a generous grinding of black pepper. Garnish with parsley. Serve with triangles of salt-free bread or salt-free pita pockets.

YIELD : 3 cups
SODIUM CONTENT: 16 mg. of sodium per 1/2-cup serving

ORANGE GINGER MARINADE FOR CHICKEN

INGREDIENTS
- 6-oz. can frozen orange juice concentrate
- 1/4 c. vegetable oil
- 2 tbsp. lemon juice
- 2 tsp. finely minced garlic
- 1 tsp. ground ginger
- 1 tbsp. finely chopped parsley

- 2 tsp. Bell's seasoning or 1/2 tsp. each of rosemary, oregano, sage, marjoram, and thyme

DIRECTIONS:

1. Thaw the orange juice concentrate, then pour it into a large bowl. Add all the other ingredients and stir to combine. To prepare chicken for the grill or broiler, immerse chicken pieces in the marinade and allow to stand for a few hours in the refrigerator, then baste them with the marinade as they cook. To maximize the flavor of the marinade, cut boneless chicken breasts into 1-inch chunks before marinating and cook them on skewers.

YIELD : 1 cup of marinade
SODIUM CONTENT: 3 mg. of sodium per 1/4 cup

BALSAMIC VINEGAR AND MUSTARD MARINADE

INGREDIENTS

- 1/2 c. balsamic vinegar
- 1/2 c. olive oil
- 2 tbsp. salt-free Dijon mustard
- 2 cloves garlic, minced freshly ground black pepper to taste

DIRECTIONS:

1. Put the vinegar, oil, and mustard in a bowl and stir with a whisk until the oil and vinegar emulsify and the mustard is evenly distributed. Stir in the minced garlic and pepper

2. If you are going to grill a steak, place it in a shallow baking dish and pour the marinade over it. After it has soaked for an hour, turn it over and let it soak for another hour. Use the marinade to baste the steak as it cooks on the grill. To maximize the flavor of the marinade, cut the meat into 1 1/2-inch cubes and grill them on skewers. If you like, you can alternate the pieces of meat with cherry tomatoes, whole mushrooms, and pieces of onion and green pepper.

YIELD : 1 cup of marinade
SODIUM CONTENT: 15 mg. of sodium per 1/4-cup serving

PEANUT DIPPING SAUCE

INGREDIENTS

- 2 tbsp. plus 2 tsp. brown sugar
- 1/4 c. salt-free rice wine vinegar or white wine vinegar
- 2 tbsp. salt-free peanut butter
- 2 tbsp. salt-free tomato paste
- 2 tbsp. water

- 1 large clove garlic, chopped
- 1/4 c. coconut milk

DIRECTIONS:

1. Put all of the ingredients except the coconut milk in a blender or food processor and blend until smooth and creamy. Transfer to a bowl and stir in the coconut milk. Keep the sauce refrigerated if you are not going to use it right away.

YIELD: 1 cup of sauce
 SODIUM CONTENT: 3 mg. of sodium per tablespoon

ORANGE DIPPING SAUCE

INGREDIENTS

- 3 tbsp. water
- 3 tbsp. dry vermouth, sherry, or white wine
- 1 shallot, chopped
- 1 clove garlic, chopped
- 2 tsp. chopped fresh ginger
- 1 tbsp. frozen orange juice concentrate
- 1 tbsp. salt-free tomato paste
- 3 tbsp. coconut milk

DIRECTIONS:

1. Put all of the ingredients except the coconut milk in a blender or food processor and blend until smooth and creamy. Transfer to a bowl and stir in the coconut milk. Keep the sauce refrigerated if you are not going to use it right away.

YIELD: 3/4 cup of sauce
 SODIUM CONTENT: 3 mg. of sodium per tablespoon

BASIL MAYONNAISE

INGREDIENTS

- 1/4 c. salt-free pasteurized egg whites
- 2 tsp. white wine vinegar
- 1 tsp. lemon juice
- 1 tsp. salt-free Dijon mustard
- 1 medium clove garlic, minced
- 1/4 tsp. sugar
- 6 fresh basil leaves, chopped
- 3/4 c. mild olive oil

DIRECTIONS:
1. Combine the egg whites, vinegar, lemon juice, mustard, garlic, sugar, and basil in a blender. Pulse a few times to combine. Then turn the blender on to high speed and add the oil in a thin stream through the hole in the lid. Close the cover completely and allow the blender to continue running until the mayonnaise firms up, about 2 minutes. You may want to stop the blending after a minute or so and use a rubber scraper to push mayonnaise down from the sides.

YIELD : 1 cup of mayonnaise
SODIUM CONTENT: 8 mg. of sodium per tablespoon

GARLIC MAYONNAISE

- **Ingredients**
- 1 medium clove garlic, chopped
- 1/4 c. salt-free pasteurized egg whites
- 1 tsp. white wine vinegar
- 1 tsp. lemon juice
- 1 tsp. salt-free Dijon mustard
- freshly ground black pepper to taste
- 3/4 c. fresh, high-quality olive oil

DIRECTIONS:
1. Combine the garlic, egg whites, vinegar, lemon juice, mustard, and pepper in a blender. Pulse a few times to combine. Then turn the blender on to high speed and add the oil in a thin stream through the hole in the lid. Close the cover completely and allow the blender to continue running until the mayonnaise firms up, about 2 minutes. You may want to stop the blending after a minute or so and use a rubber scraper to push mayonnaise down from the sides.

YIELD : 1 cup of mayonnaise
SODIUM CONTENT: 8 mg. of sodium per tablespoon

SUN-DRIED TOMATO MAYONNAISE

INGREDIENTS
- 4 halves of salt-free sun-dried tomatoes
- 1/4 c. salt-free pasteurized egg whites
- 1 tsp. white wine vinegar
- 2 tsp. lemon juice
- 3/4 c. mild olive oil

DIRECTIONS:

1. Put the halves of tomato in a small bowl, cover with boiling water, and allow to stand for 20 minutes or until soft. Combine the egg whites, vinegar, and lemon juice in a food processor. Drain the sun-dried tomatoes and use scissors or sharp knife to cut them into small pieces and drop them into the mixture as well, then pulse a few times to combine. Turn the blender on to high speed and add the oil in a thin stream through the hole in the lid. Close the cover completely and allow the blender to continue running until the mayonnaise firms up, about 2 minutes. You may want to stop the blending after a minute or so and use a rubber scraper to push mayonnaise down from the sides. Don't worry if some flecks of sun-dried tomato remain; they look fine and add tiny bursts of flavor.

YIELD: 1 cup of mayonnaise
SODIUM CONTENT: 5 mg. of sodium per tablespoon

RASPBERRY MAYONNAISE

INGREDIENTS
- 12 fresh raspberries
- 1/4 c. salt-free pasteurized egg whites
- 2 tsp. lemon juice
- 1 tbsp. sugar
- 1 c. mild olive oil

DIRECTIONS:
1. If the raspberries have a lot of seeds, seed them by pushing them through a strainer, capturing the juice and flesh in a bowl. Combine the egg whites, lemon juice, sugar, and seeded raspberries in a blender, then pulse a few times to combine. Turn the blender on to high speed and add the oil in a thin stream through the hole in the lid. Close the cover completely and allow the blender to continue running until the mayonnaise firms up, about 2 minutes. You may want to stop the blending after a minute or so and use a rubber scraper to push mayonnaise down from the sides.

YIELD: 1 1/4 cups
SODIUM CONTENT: 4 mg. of sodium per tablespoon

CRANBERRY CONSERVE

- **Ingredients**
- 12-oz. package fresh cranberries
- 1 c. water
- 1 c. sugar
- 1/2 c. raisins
- 1/4 c. orange pieces

- 1 c. shelled walnuts

DIRECTIONS:

1. Put the cranberries and water in a saucepan; bring to a boil and cook until the cranberry skins pop. Add the sugar, raisins, and orange pieces, and boil gently for 15 minutes. Stir in the nuts and allow to cool. Serve at room temperature with chicken or turkey.

YIELD : Serves 6
SODIUM CONTENT: 5 mg. of sodium per serving

HOLIDAY CRANBERRY SAUCE

INGREDIENTS

- 12-oz. package fresh cranberries
- 3/4 c. water
- 1 1/4 c. sugar
- 1/4 c. tarragon vinegar (or 1/4 c. white wine vinegar and 2 tsp. dry tarragon)
- 1/2 tsp. allspice
- 1 c. mixed dried fruit (apples, apricots, peaches, raisins) cut into small pieces

DIRECTIONS:

1. Put the cranberries in a saucepan, add the water, bring to a boil and cook until the cranberry skins pop.
2. Stir in the rest of the ingredients and bring to a boil over moderate heat. Reduce the heat to low and simmer for about 10 minutes, stirring constantly. Allow to cool before serving.

YIELD : Serves 6
SODIUM CONTENT: 5 mg. of sodium per servin

ALL-PURPOSE VEGETABLE STOCK

INGREDIENTS

- olive oil
- 1 large onion, sliced
- 4 carrots, peeled and cut into 1-inch pieces
- 4 stalks celery, cut into 1-inch pieces
- 1 bunch fresh thyme or 1 tbsp. dried thyme
- 1 bunch fresh sage or 1 tbsp. dried sage
- 1 bunch parsley
- freshly ground pepper to taste
- 4 quarts water

DIRECTIONS:

1. In a stockpot, heat a little oil to medium heat and add the onion, carrot, and celery. Cook for 10 minutes, stirring occasionally, then add all the other ingredients except the water. Allow to cook for another 5 minutes, then add the water and bring to a boil. Reduce the heat and simmer for 1 1/2 hours. Turn off the heat and allow the stock to cool. Strain before using. To save, pour 1- to 2-cup portions into resealable plastic bags and freeze.

YIELD: About 12 cups

SODIUM CONTENT: 21 mg. of sodium per cup

DOUBLE CHICKEN SOUP

INGREDIENTS

- 3 to 4 lbs. of chicken drumsticks and thighs
- 16 c. (1 gallon) cold water
- 6 sprigs fresh thyme
- 1 bunch fresh parsley, washed
- 1 tbsp. whole peppercorns
- 2 bay leaves
- 1 medium onion, peeled and halved
- cheesecloth
- 3 large carrots, peeled and quartered
- 2 half chicken breasts, bones in

DIRECTIONS:

1. Wash the chicken drumsticks and thighs and remove the skin and all visible fat. Put the cold water in a stockpot and place on high heat. Add the drumsticks and thighs and the thyme to the cold water and bring to a boil. Let the chicken boil for 1 minute, then reduce the heat so that the bubbles just break the surface of the liquid. Skim the top of the stock to get rid of the fat that accumulates as it boils off the chicken. Wrap the parsley, peppercorns, bay leaves, and onion in the cheesecloth and tie off the top with string. Add the cheesecloth bundle and the carrots to the pot. Allow the stock to simmer, covered, for 3 to 4 hours, periodically skimming the fat off the top as it accumulates.

2. Let the stock cool and strain it through a colander lined with cheesecloth. Discard the chicken, cheesecloth bundle, and carrots. Now return the stock to its original pot; add the chicken breasts, bring to a boil, reduce the heat, and allow to simmer for 2 hours. After the soup has cooked, remove the breasts. Remove the meat from the bones and return it to the soup.

YIELD: Serves 8

SODIUM CONTENT: 65 mg. of sodium per serving

TOMATO SOUP

INGREDIENTS

- 2 tbsp. unsalted butter
- 1 medium onion, chopped
- 1/2 carrot, peeled and roughly chopped
- 3 cloves garlic, chopped
- 4 c. unsalted canned tomatoes with their juice, or 4 c. chopped fresh tomatoes
- 4 fresh basil leaves, chopped, or 1 tbsp. dried basil
- 1 tsp. sugar
- freshly ground black pepper to taste
- 1 tsp. salt-free chili powder
- 2 tsp. lemon juice
- 2 c. unsalted chicken stock or broth
- milk or cream to taste (optional)
- **DIRECTIONS**

1. In a large saucepan or Dutch oven, melt the butter and cook the onion, carrot, and garlic in it for several minutes, until the onion begins to wilt. Add the tomatoes and their juice, basil, sugar, black pepper, chili powder, and lemon juice. Cook for a few minutes, then add the chicken broth or stock and bring to a boil. Reduce the heat and allow to simmer, partially covered, for about 40 minutes.
2. When the mixture has cooked, transfer it in small batches to a food processor or blender and process to a smooth liquid. Return the blended soup to the pot. At this point you can reheat and serve it as is or add milk or cream as you like before reheating.

YIELD : Serves 4
SODIUM CONTENT: 49 mg. of sodium per serving

ASPARAGUS SOUP

INGREDIENTS

- 1 large potato, peeled, quartered, and boiled until cooked through
- 2 dozen asparagus spears, trimmed and boiled or steamed until tender
- 2 to 3 c. unsalted chicken broth
- freshly ground black pepper to taste

DIRECTIONS:

1. Put the potato, asparagus, 2 cups of chicken broth, and a grinding of fresh pepper in a blender or food processor and blend well. If the soup seems too thick, add more chicken broth. The

taste and consistency will differ with the relative sizes of the potato and asparagus stalks. Strain the soup through a mesh strainer if you prefer a smooth appearance. Serve chilled or warm.

YIELD : Serves 4
SODIUM CONTENT: 30 mg. of sodium per serving

RED PEPPER SOUP

- **Ingredients**
- 4 sweet red peppers
- 1 tbsp. olive oil
- 1 clove garlic, chopped
- 1 medium onion, chopped
- 1 medium potato, peeled and cut into 1-inch pieces
- 1 c. unsalted chicken broth
- 1/2 c. milk
- sour cream or yogurt

DIRECTIONS:

1. Preheat the oven to 350 degrees. Cut the peppers in half and remove the seeds. Place the peppers cut side down on a baking sheet and brush with a little olive oil. Bake for 30 to 40 minutes, or until thoroughly tender.

2. Meanwhile, heat 1 tablespoon olive oil in a saucepan; add the garlic and onion and cook for a few minutes until the onion begins to soften. Add the potato and chicken broth. Bring to a boil, cover, reduce the heat, and simmer until the potato is tender, about 15 minutes. Add a little water if the mixture seems too dry.

3. When both the peppers and the potato mixture have cooked, cut the peppers into smaller pieces, put them in a food processor or blender, add the potato mixture, and blend until smooth. Return the mixture to the saucepan, stir in the milk, and warm over low heat to serving temperature. Pour the soup into bowls and garnish each serving with a dollop of sour cream or yogurt.

YIELD : Serves 4
SODIUM CONTENT: 40 mg. of sodium per serving

LEEK AND POTATO SOUP

INGREDIENTS

- 4 leeks, white part only
- 2 large potatoes
- 2 tbsp. unsalted butter

- 3 c. water or low-sodium chicken broth
- 3 tbsp. chopped parsley
- 2 to 3 c. whole milk
- freshly ground black pepper to taste

DIRECTIONS:

1. Clean the leeks thoroughly and chop into thin slices. Peel and dice the potatoes. Melt the butter in a large saucepan; add the leeks and cook for about 10 minutes over moderate heat, stirring to prevent burning. Add 1 cup of the water; cover and cook for a few more minutes. Then add the potatoes, parsley and the rest of the water and cook until the potatoes are tender. Add milk to taste and stir until warmed through. Add freshly ground pepper to taste.

2. The leeks and potatoes retain much of their own identity in this soup. If you prefer a creamier soup, you can transfer the mixture to a blender or food processor before adding the milk and blend until smooth. Then return to the saucepan, add milk and pepper, and heat until warmed through.

YIELD : Serves 8

SODIUM CONTENT: 73 mg. of sodium per serving with chicken broth; 60 mg. of sodium with water

SWEET CORN CHOWDER

- **Ingredients**
- 3 tbsp. unsalted butter
- 1 clove garlic, finely minced
- 1 medium onion, chopped
- 2 c. water or low-sodium chicken broth
- 11/2 c. peeled and diced potatoes
- 2 c. corn, raw, salt-free frozen, or leftover cooked without salt
- 2 c. milk
- freshly ground pepper to taste
- parsley for garnish

DIRECTIONS:

1. Melt 1 tablespoon butter in a saucepan. Add the garlic and onion and cook until the onion is translucent. Add the water or chicken broth and the potatoes. Simmer until the potatoes are cooked, about 45 minutes. Add the corn. If it is raw, allow it to simmer for a few minutes until the kernels are tender. Stir in the milk and pepper and cook on low heat until the chowder is heated through. Do not allow it to boil. Ladle into bowls and dot each bowl with a small piece of the remaining butter. Sprinkle with chopped parsley and serve immediately.

YIELD: Serves 8
SODIUM CONTENT: 20 mg. of sodium per serving with chicken broth, 9 mg. with water

MUSHROOM SOUP

INGREDIENTS

- 2 c. low-sodium chicken broth
- 2 tsp. fresh thyme leaves or 1 tsp. dried thyme
- 1 medium potato, cubed
- olive oil and unsalted butter as needed
- 1 c. chopped onion
- 2 cloves garlic, minced
- 2 c. sliced mushrooms
- 1 tbsp. lemon juice
- freshly ground black pepper to taste
- 1/2 c. red or white wine
- 1/2 c. milk
- sprigs of fresh parsley or thyme for garnish

DIRECTIONS:

1. Put the chicken broth, thyme, and potato in a saucepan and simmer until the potato is tender. Transfer to a blender or food processor and blend until smooth, then return to the saucepan. Heat a small amount of olive oil and unsalted butter in a sauté pan over medium heat and add the onion, garlic, and mushrooms. Cook for several minutes, until the onions are translucent and the mushrooms are tender. Sprinkle with the lemon juice and black pepper to taste. Add the mushroom mixture to the potato purée. Pour the wine into the sauté pan and stir with a wooden spoon to deglaze; then add to the mushroom-potato mixture. Warm the soup over low heat as you add the milk to thin it out. Serve in bowls, garnished with sprigs of fresh parsley or thyme.

YIELD: Serves 6
SODIUM CONTENT: 34 mg. of sodium per serving

CREAM OF MUSHROOM SOUP

DIRECTIONS:

- 2 tbsp. unsalted butter
- 2 1/2 c. cleaned, sliced white button mushrooms
- 1 small onion, finely chopped

- 3 tbsp. flour
- 6 c. low-sodium chicken broth
- 1 tsp. ground thyme
- 3/4 c. heavy cream

DIRECTIONS:

1. Heat a large pot to medium-high heat and add the butter. When the butter has melted, add the mushrooms and the onion. Allow to cook for 10 minutes or so, stirring occasionally, until the mushrooms start to release their liquid. Add the flour, stir to combine, then add the broth and thyme and stir well. Bring the soup to a boil, then reduce the heat to a simmer. Cook for 20 minutes. Add the cream, bring the soup back to a simmer, then turn off the heat and serve.

YIELD : Serves 6
SODIUM CONTENT: 40 mg. of sodium per serving

SQUASH AND APPLE SOUP

DIRECTIONS:

- 1 butternut squash (about 2 1/2 pounds)
- 2 medium apples
- 2 tbsp. unsalted butter
- 1/2 c. chopped onion
- 1 clove garlic, minced
- 4 c. low-sodium chicken broth
- 3 tbsp. calvados
- 1 1/2 tsp. ground cumin
- freshly ground black pepper to taste
- sour cream or yogurt

DIRECTIONS:

1. Preheat the oven to 375 degrees. Peel and seed the squash and apples and cut them into 1-inch cubes. Place the cubes in a baking pan and roast them in the oven until tender, about 1/2 an hour.
2. Melt the butter in a heavy pot; add the onion and garlic and cook until they soften. Stir the squash and apples in with the onion and garlic. Allow the mixture to cook for a few minutes, being careful not to let it burn. Then add the chicken broth, calvados, cumin, and black pepper; stir to blend.
3. Bring the mixture to a boil, reduce the heat to a simmer and cook for about 20 minutes, stirring occasionally. Remove the mixture to a blender or food processor and reduce it to a smooth purée. Return it to the pot over a low flame and keep it warm until you are ready to

serve it. To serve, spoon the soup into bowls and garnish each with a generous dollop of sour cream or yogurt.

YIELD: Serves 6
SODIUM CONTENT: 42 mg. of sodium per serving

LENTIL SOUP

INGREDIENTS
- 2 tbsp. olive oil
- 3 medium carrots, chopped
- 3 celery stalks, chopped
- 2 cloves garlic, crushed
- 1 medium onion, diced
- 1 c. chopped leftover fresh ham or pork (optional)
- 1 tsp. dried thyme or 1 tbsp. fresh thyme leaves
- freshly ground black pepper to taste
- 12 c. water
- 3 tomatoes, chopped
- 2 c. lentils, rinsed under cold water

DIRECTIONS:
1. Heat the oil to medium-high in a heavy pot or Dutch oven. Add the carrot, celery, garlic, and onion. Cook for 10 minutes until the vegetables wilt, then add the ham, thyme, and pepper. Cook for another 5 minutes, then add the water, tomato, and lentils. Bring to a boil; reduce the heat and allow the soup to simmer, covered, for 3 to 4 hours.

YIELD: Serves 8
SODIUM CONTENT: 52 mg. of sodium per serving

TUSCAN BEAN SOUP

INGREDIENTS
- 1/4 c. plus 2 tbsp. olive oil
- 1 medium onion, diced
- 1 1/2 c. salt-free freshly chopped tomatoes or 1 c. salt-free tomato sauce or purée
- 24 oz. canned salt-free navy beans or cannellini beans, drained (or 3/4 lb. dried beans soaked in water overnight)
- 2 cloves garlic, minced
- 5 c. low-sodium chicken broth
- 1 tsp. salt-free chili powder

- juice of 1/2 lemon
- 2 tbsp. fresh sage or rosemary

DIRECTIONS:
1. 6 small slices salt-free white or wheat bread, toasted and brushed with olive oil
2. Heat 2 tablespoons of oil in a large saucepan or Dutch oven; add the onion and cook until golden brown. Then add the tomatoes, beans, and garlic and stir to combine. Add the chicken broth, chili powder, and lemon juice and stir to blend. Heat to a simmer and cook for about 20 minutes if using canned beans; if using dried beans cook for about 40 minutes, or until the beans are tender.
3. Blend the soup in a blender or food processor or pass it through a food mill, then return it to the pot. Heat the rest of the olive oil in a skillet, add the sage or rosemary, and sauté for a few minutes. Stir the oil and sautéed herb into the soup mixture; bring it to a simmer once more and cook for another 20 minutes. To serve, place a slice of toasted bread in the bottom of the bowl, then pour the soup over it.

YIELD : Serves 6
SODIUM CONTENT: 35 mg. of sodium per serving

PASTA e FAGIOLI

INGREDIENTS
- 2 tbsp. olive oil
- 1 large onion, chopped
- 2 cloves garlic, finely chopped
- 2 large carrots, sliced in 1/4-inch rounds
- 1 medium zucchini, cubed
- 2 tbsp. chopped fresh basil
- 1/4 c. flat parsley leaves, tightly packed
- 1 c. fresh spinach, tightly packed
- 2 1/2 to 3 c. coarsely chopped fresh or salt-free canned tomatoes
- 15-oz. can salt-free navy beans or white kidney beans
- 1 c. salt-free chicken broth or water
- 1 tsp. dried oregano
- 1 tsp. ground cumin
- juice of 1/2 lemon
- freshly ground black pepper to taste
- 1 tbsp. white wine vinegar
- 8 oz. short pasta (spirals, elbows, bow-ties) cooked without salt

- grated unsalted Gouda or Swiss cheese (optional)

DIRECTIONS:

1. Heat the olive oil in a heavy saucepan or Dutch oven. Add the onion, garlic, and carrots and cook until the onions begin to turn brown and caramelize. Add the zucchini, basil, parsley, and spinach. Cook for a few minutes until the basil and spinach are wilted. Add the tomatoes and beans, including the liquid from the canned beans, and the chicken broth. Add the oregano, cumin, lemon juice, pepper, and vinegar, and stir to combine. Bring the mixture to a boil. Turn down the heat and allow to simmer gently for 20 to 30 minutes, until the carrots are soft and the flavors are combined.
2. To serve, put a generous serving of pasta in a large soup bowl, ladle the bean mixture over it, and sprinkle with grated cheese.

YIELD : Serves 10
SODIUM CONTENT: 4 mg. of sodium per serving

MINESTRONE

- **Ingredients**
- 1 1/2 c. whole green beans, cleaned and cut in half
- 2 tbsp. olive oil
- 2 large carrots, chopped
- 1 zucchini, chopped
- 3 tomatoes, chopped
- 10 c. salt-free chicken broth or water
- 2 c. canned salt-free kidney beans or dried kidney beans, cooked without salt
- 1 tbsp. chopped fresh basil
- freshly ground black pepper to taste
- 1/3 c. small pasta (tubes, elbows, or corkscrews)

DIRECTIONS:

1. Put the green beans in a small saucepan, cover with water, and bring to a boil. Reduce to medium heat and simmer for 20 minutes while you prepare the other ingredients. Put the oil in a large stockpot, add the vegetables and a little water or broth, cover, and cook for 10 minutes on medium to low heat. Stir occasionally to keep them from burning on the bottom. Add the rest of the water or broth, kidney beans, basil, and pepper. Turn up the heat to bring the soup to a boil, then reduce the heat and simmer for 40 minutes. Add the pasta and cook for another 12 minutes.

YIELD : Serves 8
SODIUM CONTENT: 44 mg. of sodium with chicken broth, 17 mg. with water

COLD CUCUMBER SOUP

- **Ingredients**
- 1 large cucumber, peeled
- 2 c. plain yogurt
- 1/2 c. unsalted tomato paste
- 1/2 tsp. coriander
- 1 clove garlic, minced
- mint for garnish
- freshly ground black pepper to taste

DIRECTIONS:

1. Dice the cucumber and put it in a blender or food processor. Add the rest of the ingredients except the mint and blend until smooth. Chill in the refrigerator until ready to serve, garnished with sprigs of fresh mint.

YIELD : Serves 4
SODIUM CONTENT: 76 mg. of sodium per serving

MELON SOUP WITH CALVADOS

- **Ingredients**
- 2 c. diced honeydew melon
- 2 c. diced watermelon with seeds removed
- 1 c. light cream
- 2 tbsp. calvados
- mint for garnish

DIRECTIONS:

2. Combine all the ingredients except the mint in a blender or food processor and blend until smooth. Chill until ready to serve. Garnish with sprigs of fresh mint.

YIELD : Serves 4
SODIUM CONTENT: 34 mg. of sodium per serving

MELON AND RASPBERRY SOUP

- **Ingredients**
- 1 ripe cantaloupe
- 1 c. fresh raspberries plus 4 more raspberries for garnish
- 1/2 c. orange juice
- juice of 1/2 lemon

- juice of 1/2 lime
- 4 large fresh mint leaves

DIRECTIONS:

1. Cut the melon in half, clean out the seeds, peel the halves, and cut the flesh into 1-inch pieces. Put the pieces of melon in a food processor or blender and process to create a smooth purée. Pour the melon purée into a large bowl. Put the raspberries in the food processor or blender and process to create a smooth purée. Pour this purée into a strainer and push the juice and pulp through the strainer to a small bowl in order to remove the raspberry seeds. This process should **Yield** about 1/2 cup of seedless purée (repeat with more raspberries if it comes up short).
2. Stir the raspberry purée into the melon purée, then add the orange juice, lemon juice, and lime juice, and stir to blend. To serve, ladle the soup into bowls and garnish each serving with a mint leaf and a whole raspberry.

YIELD : Serves 4
SODIUM CONTENT: 12 mg. of sodium per serving

COLE SLAW WITH FRESH HORSERADISH

- **Ingredients**
- 1/2 medium head of green cabbage
- 1/4 medium head of red cabbage
- 1/2 c. finely grated raw horseradish
- 3 tbsp. cider vinegar
- 1 tsp. sugar
- freshly ground black pepper to taste

DIRECTIONS:

1. Use a grater or food processor to reduce the cabbages to a fine grain. Put them in a bowl and stir so that the two colors are evenly distributed; then stir in the grated horseradish. Add the vinegar and stir to blend, then add the sugar and a generous grinding of pepper and stir once more. Allow to sit for at least 30 minutes before serving.

YIELD : Serves 6
SODIUM CONTENT: 19 mg. of sodium per serving

ASPARAGUS SALAD

- **Ingredients**
- 1 bunch of fresh asparagus (about a dozen spears)

- 2 hard-boiled eggs
- 3 tbsp. lemon juice
- 1/2 tsp. salt-free Dijon mustard
- freshly ground black pepper to taste
- 1 tbsp. olive oil

DIRECTIONS:

1. Trim the tough ends off the asparagus spears and boil or steam them over moderate heat until they are just tender. Remove the asparagus to cold water to prevent it cooking further and set aside. Remove the hard-boiled eggs from their shells and separate the yolks from the whites. Use a sharp knife to dice the whites and yolks as finely as possible and set them aside. Put the lemon juice, mustard, pepper, and oil in a bowl, and whisk together for the dressing.
2. Cut the tops off the asparagus and set aside. Slice the asparagus stalks into strips. Reserve 2 tablespoons of the chopped egg and put the rest in the bowl with the asparagus. Pour the dressing over the asparagus and egg mixture and toss. Garnish individual servings of the salad with asparagus tops and a sprinkling of chopped egg.

YIELD : Serves 4
SODIUM CONTENT: 50 mg. of sodium per serving

TABBOULEH

- **Ingredients**
- 1 c. bulgur wheat
- 2 c. boiling water
- 1 1/2 c. chopped parsley
- 1 c. chopped mint
- 1 c. chopped scallions
- 1 1/2 c. chopped, seeded tomatoes
- 2 carrots, steamed and cut into 1/4-inch cubes
- freshly ground black pepper to taste
- 1/3 c. lemon juice
- 1/3 c. olive oil
- 1/2 tsp. salt-free chili powder

DIRECTIONS:

1. Put the bulgur wheat in a bowl and pour the boiling water over it. Put a pot lid or plate on top of the bowl and allow to stand until the bulgur wheat has absorbed most of the water and has become tender and fluffy. Transfer the bulgur wheat to a strainer and push down on it with a rubber scraper to squeeze out any excess water.

2. Return the bulgur wheat to the bowl and add the parsley, mint, scallions, tomatoes, and carrots, stirring to distribute after each addition. Sprinkle with freshly ground pepper and stir to combine. Put the lemon juice, oil, and chili powder in a small bowl and stir to combine. Pour this mixture over the bulgur wheat mixture and toss. Chill before serving.

YIELD : Serves 8
SODIUM CONTENT: 15 mg. of sodium per serving

COUSCOUS SALAD

- **Ingredients**
- 1 1/2 c. couscous
- 1 3/4 c. boiling water
- 1 cucumber
- freshly ground black pepper to taste
- 1/2 small red onion, sliced thin
- 1 tomato, cut in half and sliced thin
- 2 tbsp. olive oil

DIRECTIONS:

1. Put the uncooked couscous in a bowl and pour the boiling water over it. Cover the bowl and allow to stand until all the water is absorbed, about 5 minutes. Remove the cover and let the couscous cool. Peel the cucumber, cut it in half lengthwise, and remove the seeds with a spoon. Dice the cucumber; place in a large bowl and add the pepper, onion, and tomato. When the couscous has cooled, fluff it with a fork and add it to the vegetables. Stir to mix, and drizzle oil over the top. Serve chilled.

YIELD : Serves 6
SODIUM CONTENT: 5 mg. of sodium per serving

CUCUMBER SALAD WITH TAHINI DRESSING

INGREDIENTS
- 3/4 c. tahini
- juice of 1 1/2 to 2 lemons
- 1 large clove garlic, finely minced
- 1/2 tsp. cumin
- 1/2 tsp. coriander
- pinch of cayenne pepper
- freshly ground black pepper to taste

- 2 cucumbers

DIRECTIONS:

1. Stir the tahini and lemon juice together until well blended. Add the rest of the ingredients except the cucumbers and stir to blend. Allow the mixture to stand at room temperature for about 30 minutes. (If you put it in the refrigerator, it will thicken up.) Peel the cucumbers and slice them into thin rounds. Put them in a large bowl, pour the dressing over them, and toss so that it is well distributed.

YIELD : Serves 4
SODIUM CONTENT: 9 mg. of sodium per serving

PICKLED CUCUMBER SALAD

INGREDIENTS

- 3 cucumbers
- 1 small red onion, sliced thin
- 2 tbsp. black peppercorns
- 3 c. white wine vinegar
- 1 tsp. sage
- juice of 1 lemon
- 1 tbsp. sugar

DIRECTIONS:

1. Peel the cucumbers and cut each in half lengthwise. Then cut across each half to create slices about 1/2-inch thick. Put all the ingredients except the cucumbers and the onion in a saucepan and bring to a boil on top of the stove. Place the cucumbers and the onion in a stainless steel bowl large enough for all the ingredients. When the vinegar mixture is at a boil, pour it over the cucumbers; cover the bowl tightly with aluminum foil or plastic wrap. When the salad cools down refrigerate it overnight. Before serving, drain off the vinegar mixture and remove the peppercorns.

YIELD : Serves 6
SODIUM CONTENT: 6 mg. of sodium per serving

ORZO AND SHRIMP SALAD

INGREDIENTS

- 1 lb. shrimp, peeled, deveined, and washed; boiled for 5 minutes
- 1/2 lb. orzo, cooked without salt in boiling water until tender (about 6 to 8 minutes)
- olive oil
- 2 fresh tomatoes, diced
- 12 basil leaves, chopped

- 1/4 c. chopped parsley
- freshly ground black pepper to taste
- juice of 1 lemon

DIRECTIONS:

1. After you have cooked and cleaned the shrimp, put them in a bowl of cold water to cool down. Drizzle the cooked orzo with olive oil, stir, and allow it to cool down as well. When the shrimp are cooled, remove them from the water to paper towels and pat them dry. Then toss all the ingredients in a large bowl until well distributed. Serve chilled.

YIELD : Serves 6
SODIUM CONTENT: 112 mg. of sodium per serving

SALADE NIÇOISE

INGREDIENTS
FOR THE SALAD:

- 2 1/2 c. cooked green beans
- 8 new potatoes cooked until fork tender and cut into quarters
- 8 plum tomatoes, quartered
- 1 small red onion, sliced thin
- 4 hard-boiled eggs, sliced
- 2 (6-oz.) cans tuna packed in water without salt

FOR THE DRESSING:

- 1/4 c. snipped parsley
- 1 tbsp. salt-free Dijon mustard
- 1 tsp. sugar
- 1/4 c. red wine vinegar
- freshly ground black pepper to taste
- 1/2 c. olive oil

DIRECTIONS:

1. Arrange the green beans, potato quarters, and tomatoes on a serving plate along with the slices of onion and hard-boiled egg. Drain the tuna and flake it over the top of the vegetables. Whisk together parsley, mustard, sugar, vinegar, and pepper. Then drizzle in the oil while continuing to whisk until it emulsifies and looks cloudy. Pour the dressing over the salad and serve.

YIELD : Serves 8
SODIUM CONTENT: 79 mg. of sodium per serving

SHRIMP SALAD WITH AVOCADO AND GRAPEFRUIT

- **Ingredients**
- 1 lb. fresh shrimp
- 1 grapefruit
- 1 avocado
- 1 red pepper, diced
- 2 tbsp. salt-free mayonnaise
- freshly ground black pepper to taste

DIRECTIONS:

1. Drop the shrimp into a pot of boiling water and cook for about 5 minutes. After the shrimp are cooked, peel off the shells and devein them. Set them aside in a bowl of ice. Cut the grapefruit in half. Peel one half, then use a sharp knife to remove sections of the flesh from the pulp; set them aside. Squeeze the other half of the grapefruit to extract the juice; set it aside. Cut the avocado in half, remove the pit, separate the flesh from the peel, and slice the flesh into sections. Pour a little of the grapefruit juice over the avocado to keep it from turning brown.
2. Combine the rest of the grapefruit juice with the diced red pepper, mayonnaise, and ground pepper in a bowl. Drain the shrimp, add them to the bowl, and stir to combine. Spoon a portion of the shrimp mixture onto each plate and place 2 or 3 avocado slices on top. Garnish the plate with the sections of grapefruit.

YIELD : Serves 6
SODIUM CONTENT: 112 mg. of sodium per serving

HEALTHY TUNA SALAD

Ingredients

FOR THE SALAD:

- 2 (6-oz.) cans tuna packed in water without salt
- 1 large carrot, peeled and grated
- 1 large cucumber, peeled, seeded, and diced
- 1/4 c. finely chopped red onion

FOR THE DRESSING:

- 1 tbsp. salt-free Dijon mustard
- 1/4 c. red wine vinegar
- 1 tsp. sugar

- 2 tbsp. finely chopped parsley
- freshly ground black pepper to taste
- 1/2 c. olive oil

DIRECTIONS:

1. Combine the four salad ingredients in a large bowl. Combine all of the dressing ingredients except the oil in a small bowl, then whisk in the oil. Combine salad and dressing to taste.

YIELD : Serves 4
 SODIUM CONTENT: 71 mg. of sodium per serving

CLASSIC TUNA SALAD

- **Ingredients**
- 2 (6-oz.) cans tuna packed in water without salt
- 1/2 c. salt-free mayonnaise
- 1/2 tsp. salt-free curry powder
- 2 tbsp. lemon juice
- freshly ground black pepper to taste

DIRECTIONS:

1. Put the tuna fish in a bowl and use a fork to mash and crumble it to an even consistency. Add the mayonnaise and stir until thoroughly blended. Then stir in the curry powder, lemon juice, and pepper. Serve on lettuce as a salad or as a filling for sandwiches on salt-free bread.

YIELD : Serves 4
 SODIUM CONTENT: 35 mg. of sodium per serving

RED POTATO SALAD WITH SWEET ONIONS

- **Ingredients**
- 10 small red potatoes
- 1 tbsp. unsalted butter
- 1 large onion, sliced
- 2 tsp. sugar
- 2 tbsp. chopped parsley
- 1 tbsp. chopped basil
- freshly ground black pepper to taste

DIRECTIONS:

1. Cut the potatoes into quarters, put them in a saucepan, cover with cold water, bring to a boil,

and cook until tender. (Or steam the potatoes until tender if you prefer.) Remove the potatoes from the heat. Cook the butter and onion in a large pan heated to medium-high heat for 10 minutes. When the onions start to brown, add the sugar and cook for another 5 minutes. Add the potatoes and the herbs to the pan, season with pepper, toss, and serve warm.

YIELD: Serves 6
SODIUM CONTENT: 12 mg. of sodium per serving

WARM NEW POTATO AND SHIITAKE MUSHROOM SALAD

- **Ingredients**
- 10 new potatoes
- 2 tbsp. olive oil
- 8 shiitake mushrooms, sliced
- juice of 1/2 lemon
- freshly ground black pepper to taste
- 1 shallot, minced
- 2 cloves garlic, diced
- 2 tbsp. chopped parsley

DIRECTIONS:

1. Wash (but don't peel) the potatoes, then cut them into quarters. Put them in a pot, cover with cold water, bring to a boil, and cook until tender. Remove the potatoes from the heat and drain. Heat olive oil in a large sauté pan over high heat. Add the mushrooms to the pan and cook for 6 minutes, then sprinkle with the lemon juice and black pepper. Add the shallot and garlic, stir to combine, and cook for another minute. Then add the potatoes and parsley; allow it all to warm through and serve.

YIELD: Serves 4
SODIUM CONTENT: 19 mg. of sodium per serving

GREEN BEAN AND SWEET POTATO SALAD

- **Ingredients**
- 2 lbs. green beans, cleaned and cut into thirds
- juice of 1/2 lemon
- 1 tbsp. unsalted Dijon mustard
- 1/4 c. red wine vinegar

- 1 tsp. sugar
- 1/4 c. chopped parsley
- freshly ground black pepper to taste
- 1/2 c. olive oil
- 1 large sweet potato, peeled, diced, and boiled until tender

DIRECTIONS:

1. Steam the green beans until tender, about 6 minutes. Remove from the pan and immerse in a bowl of cold water mixed with the lemon juice. Combine the mustard, vinegar, sugar, parsley, and black pepper in a small mixing bowl. Then drizzle in the olive oil while whisking constantly to create a creamy, blended dressing. Drain the green beans and toss with the cooked sweet potatoes in a large serving bowl. Pour the dressing over the top and stir gently to distribute. Chill the salad for an hour before serving.

YIELD : Serves 6
SODIUM CONTENT: 23 mg. of sodium per serving

POTATO AND EGG SALAD

- **Ingredients**
- 4 large potatoes, peeled and boiled
- 6 hard-boiled eggs
- 1 medium onion, chopped
- 3 tbsp. olive oil
- 2 tbsp. balsamic vinegar
- freshly ground pepper to taste
- 2 tbsp. chopped parsley

DIRECTIONS:

1. Cut the potatoes and eggs into thin slices and combine in a serving bowl. Add the chopped onion and stir gently to combine. Mix the oil and vinegar together, and stir to blend. Pour this mixture over the potatoes and eggs and stir to distribute it evenly. Add the pepper and stir once more. Sprinkle the parsley over the salad and serve.

YIELD : Serves 8
SODIUM CONTENT: 56 mg. of sodium per serving

HEALTHY POTATO SALAD

- **Ingredients**
- 8 to 10 new potatoes, boiled until tender
- juice of 1/2 lemon

- 1/4 c. olive oil
- 2 tbsp. finely chopped dill
- freshly ground black pepper to taste

DIRECTIONS:
1. When the potatoes are cooked, put them in a colander, run cold water over them, and drain; set aside to cool completely. Whisk together the lemon juice, oil, and dill. Cut the cooled potatoes into quarters and toss with the dressing. Sprinkle with freshly ground pepper and serve.

YIELD : Serves 4
SODIUM CONTENT: 12 mg. of sodium per serving

CLASSIC EGG SALAD

INGREDIENTS
- 6 hard-boiled eggs
- 1/3 c. salt-free mayonnaise
- 1/2 tsp. salt-free curry powder
- freshly ground black pepper to taste

DIRECTIONS:
1. Peel the eggs, put them in a mixing bowl, and use a fork to mash them up. Add the mayonnaise and stir to blend, followed by the curry powder and black pepper. Serve on lettuce as a salad or as filling for a sandwich on salt-free bread.

YIELD : Serves 4
SODIUM CONTENT: 92 mg. of sodium per serving

CHICKEN SALAD IN RADICCHIO LEAVES

- **Ingredients**
- 2 chicken breasts
- 1 tbsp. olive oil
- 3 tbsp. salt-free mayonnaise
- 1 orange
- 1 yellow sweet pepper
- 1 head of radicchio
- fresh parsley or cilantro for garnish

DIRECTIONS:

1. Brush the chicken breasts with the oil and broil until done. Allow them to cool completely. In a mixing bowl, combine the mayonnaise and the juice of half the orange, mixing well. Then cut up the chicken into bite-sized pieces, dice the pepper, and add them to the bowl. Peel the other half of the orange, and use a sharp knife to remove the flesh from the pulp between sections. Stir the orange into the salad. Arrange curved leaves of the radicchio so that they form a cup on each plate, fill with the salad, and garnish with sprigs of fresh parsley or cilantro.

YIELD: Serves 4
SODIUM CONTENT: 86 mg. of sodium per serving

CHICKEN SALAD WITH MANGO DRESSING

Ingredients
FOR THE SALAD:
- 2 boneless chicken breasts
- 2 mangoes, peeled, flesh cut off the seed, and diced
- 12 honeydew melon balls
- 12 cantaloupe melon balls
- radicchio leaves for garnish

FOR THE VINAIGRET TE:
- 1 mango
- 2 tbsp. white wine vinegar
- 1 tsp. sesame oil
- 1 tsp. olive oil
- 2 tbsp. white wine

DIRECTIONS:
1. Poach the chicken breasts in water for 20 to 30 minutes, until cooked through. Let cool and cut into bite-sized pieces.
2. To prepare the vinaigrette, peel the mango and remove the pit, cut into cubes, put in a blender, and blend until smooth. Add the vinegar, oils, and wine, and blend to incorporate. Put in the refrigerator to chill.
3. Toss together the chicken pieces, diced mango, and melon balls. When the dressing is chilled pour it over the salad and toss. Garnish each serving with a leaf of radicchio.

YIELD: Serves 4
SODIUM CONTENT: 90 mg. of sodium per serving

CLASSIC CHICKEN SALAD

INGREDIENTS

- 2 c. diced chicken; roasted, broiled, or sautéed without salt; skin and bones removed
- 1/2 c. salt-free mayonnaise
- 1/2 tsp. salt-free chili powder
- 1 tsp. lemon juice
- **DIRECTIONS**

1. Put the diced chicken in a bowl; add the rest of the ingredients and stir to combine well. Serve as a filling for sandwiches on salt-free bread, or as a salad by placing a scoop of the chicken mixture on a large leaf of romaine or red leaf lettuce, garnished with a sprig of parsley.

YIELD : Serves 4;
SODIUM CONTENT: 83 mg. of sodium per serving

AVOCADO AND BEAN SALAD

INGREDIENTS

- 2 avocados, peeled, pitted, and diced
- 15-ounce can unsalted pinto, black, or kidney beans
- 8 cherry tomatoes, halved
- 1 shallot, minced
- juice of 1/2 lemon
- freshly ground pepper to taste

DIRECTIONS:

1. Place the first four ingredients in a bowl and stir to combine. Sprinkle with the lemon juice and pepper, and toss well. Serve chilled.

YIELD : Serves 4
SODIUM CONTENT: 31 mg. of sodium per serving

BLACK BEAN SALAD

Ingredients

FOR THE SALAD:

- 2 c. cooked black beans or 15-ounce can salt-free canned beans
- 1 medium onion, diced
- 1 sweet red pepper, white membrane removed, seeded, and diced
- 2 c. salt-free frozen or fresh corn

- 1 tbsp. chopped fresh cilantro leaves

FOR THE DRESSING:
- 1/4 c. olive oil
- 1/4 c. balsamic vinegar
- 1 tbsp. unsalted Dijon mustard
- freshly ground black pepper to taste

DIRECTIONS:
1. If using canned beans, drain off their liquid. Combine the beans, onion, pepper, corn, and cilantro in a large bowl. Mix the dressing ingredients together in a small bowl and stir with a whisk until thoroughly blended. Pour the dressing over the bean mixture and stir to distribute it evenly.

YIELD: Serves 6
SODIUM CONTENT: 19 mg. of sodium per serving

LENTIL SALAD

- **Ingredients**
- 1 1/2 c. dried lentils
- 1 medium tomato, chopped
- 2 tbsp. chopped fresh parsley
- 1 tbsp. chopped fresh tarragon
- 1 tbsp. balsamic vinegar
- 2 tbsp. olive oil
- freshly ground black pepper to taste
- 1 medium red onion, chopped fine

DIRECTIONS:
1. Boil the lentils in unsalted water for 35 minutes or until tender. When the lentils are cooked through, place them in a large serving bowl. Add the rest of the ingredients and toss to combine. Serve chilled.

YIELD: Serves 6
SODIUM CONTENT: 17 mg. of sodium per serving

TUSCAN BEAN SALAD

- **Ingredients**
- 2 cans salt-free white beans or 2 c. dried navy beans
- 3 tbsp. chopped parsley
- 2 tbsp. chopped basil

- 1 tbsp. chopped sage
- freshly ground black pepper to taste
- juice of 1/2 lemon
- 2 tbsp. olive oil

DIRECTIONS:

1. If you are using dried beans, wash them in cool water and boil for 20 minutes. Then drain and boil again until they are tender; this could take up to 2 hours. While the beans are simmering you can flavor them with black pepper and a lemon wedge, fresh herbs, or a couple of garlic cloves.
2. Drain the beans (whether canned or home cooked), put them in a large bowl with all the rest of the ingredients, and stir to combine. Let stand for 1 hour before serving.

BROILED SEA BASS

- **Ingredients**
- 1/4 c. olive oil
- juice of 1/2 lemon
- freshly ground black pepper to taste
- 2 tbsp. chopped fresh parsley
- 1 tbsp. chopped fresh tarragon
- 2 cloves garlic, crushed
- 4 (8-oz.) pieces of sea bass cut in thick fillets

DIRECTIONS:

1. Mix together all the ingredients except the fish in a shallow dish. Add the fish and turn to coat with the oil-herb mixture. Allow the fish to marinate for 20 to 30 minutes. In the meantime heat the broiler and make sure the rack in the oven is 8 to 10 inches away from the heat source.
2. After the fish has marinated, remove it from the oil and place it in an ovenproof baking dish. It's not necessary to drain off all the oil—that's where the flavor is. Put the fish under the broiler for 8 minutes, checking occasionally to make sure it doesn't burn. The fish is ready when cooked through and just beginning to brown on top.

YIELD : Serves 4
SODIUM CONTENT: 157 mg. of sodium per serving

STRIPED BASS WITH BRAISED TOMATO

- **Ingredients**

- 2 (12-oz.) fillets of striped sea bass
- freshly ground black pepper to taste
- 2 tbsp. olive oil
- 1 small shallot, chopped
- 3 cloves garlic, sliced
- 2 medium tomatoes, chopped
- 2 tbsp. chopped parsley
- 1 tsp. fresh dill
- 5 large basil leaves, roughly chopped
- 1/3 c. white wine
- juice of 1/2 lemon

DIRECTIONS:
1. Rinse the fish fillets in cool water and pat dry. Cut each fillet in half to create two squarish pieces. Season with pepper and set aside. Heat 2 tablespoons olive oil in a sauté pan; add the fish, skin side down. Cook for 4 minutes, shaking the pan to prevent sticking. Remove the fish from the pan. Add the shallot and garlic to the pan, season with pepper, and cook for 6 minutes. Add the tomatoes and all the herbs, stirring, and cook for another 5 minutes. Add the white wine and lemon juice and reseason with black pepper. Reduce heat to a simmer, cover, and allow to cook for 12 to 15 minutes.

    Return the fish to the pan, skin side down, cover the pan, and cook for 8 minutes. Put a piece of fish on each plate with a dollop of tomatoes. Use a spoon to drizzle some of the pan juices around the fish.

YIELD : Serves 4
SODIUM CONTENT: 126 mg. of sodium per serving

BAKED WHOLE RED SNAPPER OR SEA BASS

INGREDIENTS
- 1 small onion
- 1 lemon
- 1 whole fresh fish, scaled and cleaned
- freshly ground black pepper to taste
- 10 sprigs of fresh parsley
- 1/2 c. white wine

DIRECTIONS:

1. Preheat the oven to 400 degrees. Peel the onion and slice it very thin. Slice thin cross sections of the lemon. Cut slices crosswise across the top side of the fish to make serving sized pieces. Place the fish in an ovenproof baking dish and sprinkle with black pepper. Distribute the onion, lemon slices, and parsley over the fish and pour the wine around it. Bake in the oven for 25 minutes or until the fish flakes when poked. When the fish has cooked, the slices should lift off the bone easily. Then remove the bone and cut pieces from the bottom side of the fish. Avoid serving pieces containing small bones near the head and fins.

YIELD : Serves 2 or more
SODIUM CONTENT: 124 mg. of sodium per 6 ounces of fish

CAJUN SWORDFISH STEAKS

- **Ingredients**
- 1/2 tsp. dried basil
- 1/2 tsp. dried parsley
- 1/4 tsp. dried oregano
- 1 tbsp. paprika
- pinch of cumin
- pinch of cayenne pepper
- freshly ground pepper to taste
- 2 (8-oz.) swordfish steaks
- 1 tbsp. olive oil

DIRECTIONS:
1. Mix all the spices together in a bowl. Wash and dry the fish. Sprinkle the spice mixture evenly over one side of the fish. Allow to sit for 10 minutes. Heat the oil in a nonstick pan and reduce the heat to medium. Add the fish, seasoned side down, and cook for 5 minutes. Turn the fish over and continue cooking for about 3 more minutes, until it is cooked through.

YIELD : Serves 2
SODIUM CONTENT: 125 mg. of sodium per serving

BAKED FLOUNDER WITH FENNEL SAUCE

- **Ingredients**
- 2 fennel bulbs, cubed
- 1/4 c. white wine
- 1/2 c. sour cream or quark
- 2 tbsp. lemon juice

- 4 (6-oz.) flounder fillets
- 1 tbsp. fennel seeds
- 1 clove garlic, minced

DIRECTIONS:

1. Steam the fennel until tender, then purée in a blender or food processor. Add the wine, sour cream or quark, and 1 tablespoon lemon juice, and stir to combine. Set the sauce aside.

2. Preheat the oven to 350 degrees. Rinse the flounder fillets and pat dry. Use an electric spice grinder or a mortar and pestle to pulverize the fennel seeds. Combine the seeds, minced garlic, and 1 tablespoon of lemon juice and rub it gently into the surface of the fish. Put the fish fillets in a lightly buttered ovenproof dish and cover with the fennel sauce. Bake until the fish is cooked through, about 1/2 hour.

YIELD: Serves 4

SODIUM CONTENT: 178 mg. of sodium per serving

FLOUNDER POACHED IN TOMATO AND WINE

- **Ingredients**
- 3 oz. salt-free tomato paste
- 1/2 c. water
- 3/4 c. white wine
- juice of 1/2 lemon
- 1 tbsp. dried basil or 2 tbsp. chopped fresh basil leaves
- 4 (6-oz.) flounder fillets
- freshly ground black pepper to taste
- sprigs of parsley for garnish

DIRECTIONS:

1. Stir the tomato paste, water, wine, and lemon juice together in a bowl until well blended, then pour into a skillet large enough to accommodate the fish fillets lying flat. Heat briefly and add the basil. Place the fish fillets in the skillet so that they are partially covered by the liquid; sprinkle evenly with the pepper. When the liquid begins to simmer, turn down the heat, cover, and cook until the fish is cooked through, about 10 minutes. Remove the fish to a warm platter, then turn up the heat and allow the liquid to cook down for a minute or so. Pour enough of the liquid over the fish fillets to cover them, garnish with fresh parsley, and serve immediately. Pour the remainder of the liquid into a bowl and serve as additional sauce for the fish.

YIELD: Serves 4

SODIUM CONTENT: 151 mg. of sodium per serving

FLOUNDER BAKED IN PARCHMENT

INGREDIENTS

- 6-oz. fresh flounder fillet
- 1/2 c. finely diced leeks
- 1 small shallot, finely diced
- 1 tbsp. olive oil
- 1/2 c. carrots cut into julienne strips
- 4 string beans cut into thin strips
- 2 sprigs of fresh thyme
- 2 tbsp. white wine
- freshly ground black pepper to taste

DIRECTIONS:

1. Preheat the oven to 400 degrees. Rinse the fish and pat dry. Combine the diced leeks and shallot in a small bowl. Cut a sheet of parchment paper about 12 inches wide and 15 inches long. Fold in half the long way to make a crease. Using your fingers or a pastry brush, spread the olive oil over half of the paper (on one side of the crease), to within an inch of the outside edges. Be sure to leave the edges dry.
2. Spread a few pieces of carrot and string beans as well as a third of the leek-shallot mixture on the oiled paper and place the fish fillet on top. Pile the rest of the vegetables on top of the fish and place the thyme across them. Sprinkle with the wine and pepper.
3. Fold the dry half of the parchment over the fish and vegetables and fold the edges tightly, starting at a corner by the crease, to create a semicircular pouch. Fold the edges over two or three times so that they stay together. Put the pouch on a baking sheet, place it in the oven, and bake for 10 to 12 minutes, until the fish is cooked through.

YIELD : Serves 1

SODIUM CONTENT: 164 mg. of sodium per serving

OVEN-ROASTED SALMON WITH TOMATOES AND ASPARAGUS

- **Ingredients**
- 2 lemons
- 4 (6-oz.) salmon steaks
- 8 asparagus spears, trimmed
- 2 medium tomatoes, sliced

- 4 fresh basil leaves
- 1/4 c. white wine
- freshly ground black pepper to taste
- 2 tbsp. chopped parsley

DIRECTIONS:

1. Preheat the oven to 375 degrees. Slice one of the lemons into thin circles and distribute them over the bottom of an ovenproof baking dish or pan large enough to hold all the fish. Add the steaks and arrange the asparagus, tomato slices, and basil leaves around them. Then add the wine and sprinkle everything with the pepper and parsley. Roast in the oven until the fish is cooked through, 12 to 16 minutes, depending on the size of the steaks. Serve with slices of the second lemon.

YIELD: Serves 4
SODIUM CONTENT: 120 mg. of sodium per serving

SALMON IN A BASIL BUTTER SAUCE

- **Ingredients**
- 4 (6-oz.) salmon fillets
- 1 c. water
- juice of 1/2 lemon
- 4 tbsp. unsalted butter
- 1 shallot, finely diced
- 1 clove garlic, finely diced
- 8 fresh basil leaves, roughly chopped
- sprigs of basil for garnish

DIRECTIONS:

1. Rinse the fish in cold water and remove any bones. Put the fish in a large sauté pan; add the water and lemon juice, and poach the fish in simmering liquid until it has turned pink all the way through, about 8 to 10 minutes. Meanwhile, in a small saucepan, combine butter, shallot, and garlic, and cook over low heat only until the butter has melted—make sure not to brown the butter. Then stir in the basil.

2. When the salmon is done, remove each fillet to a plate and spoon the butter sauce over and around it. Garnish each fillet with a sprig of basil leaves. Serve hot.

YIELD: Serves 4
SODIUM CONTENT: 114 mg. of sodium per serving

GRILLED SALMON STEAKS WITH

HERBED BUTTER

- **Ingredients**
- 4 tbsp. (1/2 stick) unsalted butter, softened
- 2 tbsp. finely chopped parsley
- 1 tbsp. finely chopped basil
- 2 sage leaves, finely chopped
- juice of 1/2 lemon
- freshly ground black pepper to taste
- 4 (8- to 10-oz.) salmon steaks

DIRECTIONS:

1. Put the butter in a bowl; add the herbs, lemon juice, and pepper, and stir to blend. Coat each steak liberally with the herbed butter. Allow to marinate while you prepare the charcoal or gas grill. When the grill reaches medium-high heat, put the steaks on it and cook about 4 minutes on one side; turn once and cook 3 minutes more, then remove.

YIELD : Serves 4
 SODIUM CONTENT: 187 mg. of sodium per serving

COLD POACHED SALMON WITH CUCUMBER DILL SAUCE

Ingredients

FOR THE FISH:

- 1 large salmon fillet, about 24 oz.
- water to cover the bottom of the pan, about 1 1/2 cups
- 6 peppercorns
- 1 bay leaf
- 1 tbsp. lemon juice

FOR THE SAUCE:

- 1 c. plain yogurt or sour cream
- 1/2 c. peeled and diced cucumber
- 1 tbsp. lemon juice
- 2 tbsp. finely chopped fresh dill

DIRECTIONS:

1. Check the salmon fillet for bones and remove any you find. Bring the water, peppercorns, bay leaf, and lemon juice to a boil in a skillet large enough to hold the fillet lying flat. The

liquid should be about 1/2-inch deep, enough to partially cover the fish. Place the fish in the liquid. When it returns to a boil, turn down the heat so that it continues to simmer gently. Cover loosely and poach for about 10 minutes, or until the fish is tender and cooked through. Allow to cool, then put in the refrigerator to chill.

2. To make the sauce, put the yogurt or sour cream and cucumber in a blender or food processor and blend until the cucumber is puréed. Add the lemon juice and dill and pulse several times to mix.

3. To serve, put the fish on a platter, pour some of the sauce over it, and garnish with a few whole sprigs of dill. Serve the rest of the sauce in a bowl.

YIELD : Serves 4
SODIUM CONTENT: 137 mg. of sodium per serving

SALMON CAKES

INGREDIENTS

- 1-lb. salmon fillet, diced very small
- 1 tsp. chopped fresh dill
- 1 tbsp. chopped parsley
- 1 tbsp. salt-free Dijon mustard
- 2 tbsp. finely diced sweet red pepper
- 1 c. salt-free bread crumbs
- 1 tbsp. unsalted butter

DIRECTIONS:

1. Combine all the ingredients except the bread crumbs and butter in a bowl and mix them together with your fingers until well blended. Then begin adding bread crumbs a small amount at a time, continuing to mix them in by hand, until the mixture thickens enough so that you can form it into balls that hold together. Each cake should be the size of a large meatball, slightly flattened. Put the cakes on a plate, cover loosely with plastic wrap and refrigerate for a 1/2 hour.

2. Heat the butter in a nonstick skillet to medium heat; add the cakes and cook, turning once, 3 to 4 minutes per side, taking care not to let them burn. The cakes will be fragile; it is all right to let them fall apart a bit as they cook.

YIELD : Serves 6
SODIUM CONTENT: 62 mg. of sodium per serving

SEARED SCALLOPS WITH SPRING VEGETABLES

- **Ingredients**

- 1 c. baby carrots, peeled and washed
- 1 c. green beans washed and cut into 2-inch strips
- 1 c. fresh baby spinach, washed
- 1 red pepper, seeded and cut into thin strips
- vegetable oil
- 12 large sea scallops, cleaned and rinsed
- juice of 1 lemon

DIRECTIONS:

1. Steam the carrots until just tender; do the same with the green beans. Toss the carrots, raw spinach leaves, green beans, and red pepper in a bowl and set aside. Heat a small amount of oil over high heat in a nonstick sauté pan. Make sure the scallops are completely dry. Place them in the pan, season with black pepper, and cook for 3 minutes on each side, until golden brown. Discard any that burn. Remove the scallops from the pan to a paper towel in order to drain off excess oil. For each serving, take a handful of the vegetables and put it on a plate, place three scallops on top of them, and drizzle with some of the lemon juice.

YIELD : Serves 4
SODIUM CONTENT: 151 mg. per serving

MUSHROOM, TOMATO, AND SHRIMP OMELET

INGREDIENTS

- 2 tbsp. unsalted butter
- 2 c. sliced mushrooms
- freshly ground black pepper to taste
- 8 eggs
- 1/2 c. milk
- 2 medium tomatoes, diced
- 1/2 lb. popcorn shrimp, cooked without salt

DIRECTIONS:

1. Melt 1 tablespoon of butter in a skillet over medium heat. Add the mushrooms and season with pepper. Sauté until the mushrooms release their juices. Remove from the heat. Place 2 eggs in a bowl, season with pepper, add 2 tablespoons of milk and whisk until the milk, yolks, and whites are all well combined. Heat a separate nonstick pan over medium heat and add a small dab of butter. Add the egg mixture to the pan and cook until it starts to set. As it does, add one-fourth of the tomatoes, shrimp, and mushrooms, and distribute them evenly over the surface of the eggs. Finish cooking the omelet to the degree of firmness you like,

then slide half of it onto a plate and flip the pan so that the other half folds on top of it. Repeat for the other three omelets. Serve immediately.

YIELD: Serves 4
SODIUM CONTENT: 232 mg. of sodium per serving

VIII. POULTRY

CHICKEN WITH MUSTARD SAUCE

INGREDIENTS
FOR THE SAUCE:
- 1/3 c. salt-free mayonnaise
- 2 tbsp. salt-free Dijon mustard
- dash of onion powder
- dash of garlic powder
- freshly ground black pepper to taste
- 2 tbsp. chopped parsley

FOR THE CHICKEN:
- 2 whole chicken breasts (4 half breasts)
- 1/2 c. flour
- 1 tbsp. corn oil
- 1/4 c. low-sodium chicken broth

DIRECTIONS:
1. Put the ingredients for the sauce in a bowl; mix and set aside. Wash and pat the chicken breasts dry and dredge with flour. Heat the oil in a large skillet. When it is hot, slip the chicken into the skillet; brown quickly on both sides and remove. Deglaze the pan with the chicken broth (add the broth and stir to dissolve the residue on the bottom and sides of the pan), and cook until it is reduced by half. Then spoon in the sauce and stir. Add the chicken breasts and simmer for 15 to 20 minutes, or until the chicken is cooked through.

YIELD: Serves 4
SODIUM CONTENT: 125 mg. of sodium per serving

BALSAMIC GLAZED CHICKEN

- **Ingredients**
- 1/2 c. balsamic vinegar
- 2 tbsp. olive oil
- 2 cloves garlic, crushed
- 1 tsp. ground sage

- 1 dash dried thyme
- 1 shallot, minced
- freshly ground black pepper to taste
- 4-lb. roasting chicken

DIRECTIONS:

1. Combine all the ingredients except the chicken in a large bowl and stir to blend. Wash the chicken inside and out and pat dry with paper towels. Place the chicken in the bowl and spoon the marinade over it, making sure to coat the whole bird. Cover and marinate in the refrigerator for at least 3 hours, overnight if possible. Preheat the oven to 375 degrees. Place the chicken on a rack in a roasting pan and pour the marinade over it. Roast for 11/2 hours or until the juices run clear when a leg of the chicken is cut.

YIELD : Serves 6
SODIUM CONTENT: 119 mg. of sodium per serving

WHITE WINE BRAISED CHICKEN

- **Ingredients**
- olive oil
- 3 lbs. chicken pieces, washed and dried
- 1/2 c. white wine
- 2 tbsp. chopped fresh parsley
- 1/2 onion, chopped
- 4 fresh sage leaves
- 4 cloves garlic, chopped
- freshly ground black pepper to taste

DIRECTIONS:

1. Preheat the oven to 350 degrees. On top of the stove, heat an ovenproof skillet or Dutch oven large enough to hold all the ingredients. When it has reached high heat, add enough oil to coat the bottom of the pan. Add the chicken pieces skin sides down to brown, then turn to brown the other sides. When the chicken has thoroughly browned, remove the pieces and deglaze the pan with the wine (add the wine and stir to dissolve the residue on the bottom and sides of the pan). Return the chicken pieces to the pan, add the rest of the ingredients, cover, and place in the oven to bake for 45 minutes. Serve the chicken with rice and generous spoonfuls of the pan juices.

YIELD : Serves 6
SODIUM CONTENT: 100 mg. of sodium per serving

BORDEAUX BRAISED CHICKEN

- **Ingredients**
- olive oil
- 1 c. chopped onion
- 1 c. chopped carrot
- 1 c. chopped green pepper
- 3 sprigs fresh tarragon
- 3 sprigs fresh sage
- 6 stalks fresh parsley
- freshly ground black pepper to taste
- 2 c. Bordeaux wine
- 1 c. low-sodium chicken broth
- 8 small pieces of dark chicken meat (drumsticks and thighs)

DIRECTIONS:

1. Heat a pan large enough for all the ingredients to medium-high and coat the bottom with oil. Add the onion, carrot, and green pepper. Cook for about 10 minutes, stirring occasionally, then add the herbs and black pepper, and cook for another 5 minutes. Add the wine and the chicken broth; stir to blend. Cook the mixture until it is reduced by half. Add the chicken, cover, and allow to simmer very gently until the meat is falling off the bone, about 45 minutes. Remove the chicken to a serving plate. Strain the sauce and drizzle a little over the chicken, reserving the rest in a gravy boat to serve with the meat.

YIELD : Serves 4
SODIUM CONTENT: 153 mg. of sodium per serving

BAKED CHICKEN WITH APPLE CIDER AND APPLES

- **Ingredients**
- 3 lbs. chicken pieces
- 2 c. apple cider
- 1/2 c. flour
- 1 tsp. ground ginger
- 1 tsp. ground cinnamon
- freshly ground black pepper to taste
- 2 tbsp. brown sugar
- 2 medium apples

DIRECTIONS:

1. Remove the skin and fat from the chicken pieces and wash them in cold water. Put the cider in a large bowl; add the brown sugar and stir to dissolve. Add the chicken pieces, cover, and allow to marinate for a few hours or overnight.
2. Preheat the oven to 350 degrees. Combine the flour, ginger, cinnamon, and pepper in another bowl and stir to blend. Remove the chicken from the cider marinade and reserve the liquid. Dip each chicken piece in the flour mixture and coat well, then place in a baking pan and bake for 30 minutes. Core the apples, cut into thin slices, and add them to the cider marinade. Remove chicken from the baking pan and pour in the cider-apple mixture. Return chicken to the pan and bake for another 25 minutes or until the chicken is cooked through.
3. Remove the chicken pieces to a serving dish. Deglaze the pan (use a wooden spoon to scrape bits of chicken and apple from the bottom and sides) and, if necessary, cook down the cider-apple mixture to make a sauce. If it has cooked down too much already, add a little cider. Serve the chicken pieces using the cider-apple mixture as a sauce.

YIELD : Serves 6
SODIUM CONTENT: 82 mg. of sodium per serving

CHICKEN BREASTS STUFFED WITH WILD MUSHROOMS

INGREDIENTS
- 3 large button mushrooms
- 4 chanterelle mushrooms
- 4 shiitake mushrooms
- 2 to 3 tbsp. olive oil
- 1 shallot, minced
- 1 clove garlic, minced
- 2 tbsp. balsamic vinegar
- 1 tbsp. dried parsley or 2 tbsp. chopped fresh parsley
- 2 whole boneless chicken breasts (4 half breasts) pounded between plastic wrap to 1/4-inch thick
- toothpicks

DIRECTIONS:
1. Chop the mushrooms, place them in a hot sauté pan with 1 tablespoon of olive oil (use more oil if needed), and reduce to moderate heat. Cook the mushrooms for 5 minutes, then add the minced shallot, parsley, and garlic. Cook for 5 more minutes; add the vinegar and deglaze the pan by stirring until all of the residue on the bottom of the pan has dissolved in it. This should take about a minute. Remove the mushroom mixture to a plate.
2. Preheat the oven to 350 degrees. When it is cool enough to handle, spread about 2

tablespoons of the mushroom mixture on each flattened piece of chicken and roll it up. Use toothpicks to secure the roll and keep it closed. Heat 1 to 2 tablespoons of olive oil in the pan you used to prepare the mushrooms and brown the chicken on all sides. Transfer the chicken rolls to a baking dish and cook in the oven until the chicken is cooked through, about 20 minutes.

YIELD : Serves 4
SODIUM CONTENT: 83 mg. of sodium per serving

CHICKEN TENDERS

INGREDIENTS

- 1 c. all-purpose flour
- 1 tbsp. cumin or salt-free chili powder
- freshly ground black pepper to taste
- 2 whole boneless chicken breasts (4 half breasts), cut into 1-inch cubes
- vegetable oil

DIRECTIONS:

1. Combine the flour, cumin or salt-free chili powder, and pepper in a paper bag. Put the chicken cubes in the bag and shake until all the pieces are evenly coated with the flour mixture. Pour enough oil into a large skillet to cover the bottom to a depth of 1/8 inch and heat to medium-high. Drop the chicken pieces into the oil and cook for about 5 minutes on one side, then turn and cook for another 5 minutes. Remove cooked pieces to a plate lined with a paper towel so that the oil drains off. Serve with a sprinkling of lemon juice, lemon wedges, salt-free hot sauce or dipping sauces.

YIELD : Serves 4
SODIUM CONTENT: 82 mg. of sodium per serving

GRILLED LEMON CHICKEN

- **Ingredients**
- 3 whole boneless chicken breasts (6 half breasts)
- juice of 1 lemon
- freshly ground pepper to taste
- 1 tbsp. unsalted Dijon mustard
- 1/2 c. red wine vinegar
- 2 tbsp. chopped fresh parsley
- 4 basil leaves, chopped
- 1 tsp. dried oregano
- 1/4 c. olive oil

- pinch of ground sage

DIRECTIONS:

1. Make a marinade by combining all the ingredients except the chicken in a large bowl and mixing well. Wash the chicken and trim any excess fat. Put the chicken in the bowl with the marinade, turn the pieces to coat them, and put in the refrigerator to marinate for at least an hour. Prepare the charcoal or gas grill, and grill chicken pieces over medium heat until cooked through.

YIELD : Serves 6

SODIUM CONTENT: 88 mg. of sodium per serving

CHICKEN BREASTS IN A PEANUT SAUCE

INGREDIENTS

- 2 whole boneless chicken breasts, cut into 4 half breasts
- 1/4 c. brown sugar
- 1/4 c. white wine vinegar
- 1/4 c. salt-free peanut butter
- 1/4 c. salt-free tomato paste
- 2 large cloves garlic, chopped

DIRECTIONS:

1. Rinse the chicken breasts in cold water, pat dry, and place them in a shallow bowl. Whisk the rest of the ingredients together in a small bowl; pour the mixture over the chicken pieces and turn them so they are coated evenly. Marinate for at least an hour. Cook the chicken pieces under the broiler or on a charcoal grill, basting with the remainder of the marinade, until cooked through.

YIELD : Serves 4

SODIUM CONTENT: 91 mg. of sodium per serving

BROILED CHICKEN WITH MUSTARD AND HORSERADISH

INGREDIENTS

- 3 whole boneless, skinless chicken breasts, cut in half
- 2 tbsp. unsalted Dijon mustard
- 2 tbsp. salt-free mayonnaise
- 1/2 tsp. ground cumin

- 1 tsp. cider vinegar
- 2 tbsp. grated fresh horseradish or 2 tsp. salt-free prepared horseradish
- olive oil
- freshly ground black pepper to taste
- **DIRECTIONS**

1. Preheat the oven broiler. Rinse the pieces of chicken breast and dry completely with a paper towel. Combine the mustard, mayonnaise, cumin, vinegar, and 1 tablespoon of the grated horseradish (or all of the prepared horseradish) in a bowl, and stir until well blended. Use a pastry brush to coat the bottom of a shallow pan with olive oil. Place the chicken breasts in the pan, outer side down, then use a brush to add a light coating of oil to their exposed sides. Use the brush to spread the mustard-horseradish mixture on the exposed inner sides of the breasts, then turn them over and spread the mixture on the outer sides. Sprinkle with pepper and the rest of the grated horseradish. Place on the middle shelf of the oven under the broiler or on the lowest level of a separate broiler and cook until the breasts are golden brown on top and cooked through, about 15 minutes.

YIELD : Serves 6
SODIUM CONTENT: 115 mg. of sodium per serving

TANDOORI-STYLE CHICKEN

INGREDIENTS
- 3 whole boneless and skinless chicken breasts (or 6 half breasts)
- 1 pinch of saffron
- 1 tbsp. cumin
- 2 tsp. coriander
- 2 cloves garlic, crushed
- 1 c. plain yogurt

DIRECTIONS:

1. Rinse the chicken breasts, pat dry with a paper towel and cut into inch-thick strips. Mix all the spices, garlic, and yogurt together in a large bowl. Add the chicken to the bowl, cover, and allow to marinate for at least 2 hours.

2. Prepare the charcoal or gas grill; when it is at medium to medium-high heat, place the chicken pieces on it until they are cooked through, turning them from time to time so they cook evenly on all sides. This should take about 10 minutes. Serve with rice.

YIELD : Serves 6
SODIUM CONTENT: 97 mg. of sodium per serving

ROASTED PEPPERS STUFFED WITH

CHICKEN

- **Ingredients**
- 2 whole chicken breasts, cut into 4 half breasts, cleaned and trimmed of excess fat
- 1/2 c. balsamic vinegar
- 1 tbsp. olive oil
- freshly ground black pepper to taste
- 2 tbsp. diced red onion
- 2 tbsp. chopped parsley
- 1 tbsp. chopped basil
- 1 tomato, diced
- 4 sweet red peppers

DIRECTIONS:

1. Marinate the chicken for about 20 minutes in the balsamic vinegar with the oil and black pepper. Grill the chicken over a charcoal grill or sauté it on top of the stove until cooked through. When it has cooled, chop it into very small pieces and place it in a bowl. Add the onion, parsley, basil, tomato, and black pepper; stir to combine. Roast the whole peppers until tender over the charcoal grill or a gas flame, or on a baking sheet in a 350-degree oven. Remove the stems, cut off the tops, remove the seeds, and fill each pepper with a generous amount of the chicken mixture. (If the peppers won't hold their shapes, spread pieces of them on plates and cover with the chicken mix.)

YIELD : Serves 4
SODIUM CONTENT: 83 mg. of sodium per serving

CHICKEN SCALOPPINE WITH MUSHROOMS

- **Ingredients**
- 2 whole boneless chicken breasts cut into 4 half breasts
- flour for dredging
- 2 to 3 tbsp. olive oil
- 1 c. sliced mushrooms
- 2 tsp. lemon juice
- freshly ground black pepper to taste
- 1/2 c. grated low-sodium Gouda or Swiss cheese
- parsley for garnish

DIRECTIONS:
1. Dredge a piece of chicken breast in flour, then sprinkle a little more flour on a piece of waxed paper and place the chicken on it. Pound the chicken flat, to a thickness of 1/4 inch, using the bottom of a heavy skillet or pot. Repeat with the other pieces of chicken. Heat 2 tablespoons of oil in a large sauté pan; add the mushrooms and cook over medium heat to the point that they begin to wilt and give up their liquid. Sprinkle with 1 teaspoon of the lemon juice and a grinding of black pepper and stir to combine. Remove the mushrooms and put the chicken pieces in the pan, adding a bit more oil if necessary.
2. Turn up the heat and cook the chicken just until cooked on the bottom and the edges begin to turn white. Turn the chicken pieces over and place equal portions of mushrooms on top of each one, then sprinkle generously with grated cheese and with another teaspoon of lemon juice. Turn the heat down to low; cover and cook for a few more minutes until the cheese has melted and the chicken is cooked through.

YIELD : Serves 4
SODIUM CONTENT: 78 mg. of sodium per serving

TWO CHICKEN STEW

- **Ingredients**
- 2 tbsp. olive oil
- 2 medium onions, roughly chopped
- 1 bunch fresh sage (a dozen leaves or more)
- 1 bunch fresh thyme
- 1 bunch parsley
- 2 whole chickens (about 3 1/2 lbs. each)
- 4 quarts water
- 2 tbsp. whole black peppercorns
- 4 large carrots, peeled and cut into 1-inch lengths
- 10 new potatoes, quartered
- 2 medium tomatoes, diced

DIRECTIONS:
1. Heat the oil in a large pot or Dutch oven and sauté the onion and the herbs in it for about 10 minutes. Add the chickens, water, and peppercorns; bring to a boil. Turn down the heat and allow to simmer for 4 hours. Use a large spoon to skim off the fat as it collects on the surface.
2. After 4 hours, turn off the heat and allow to cool. Take the chickens out of the pot, and remove and discard the skin and fat. Separate the meat from the bones and break the meat into bite-sized pieces. Use a ladle to strain the liquid through a fine strainer or colander into a bowl, and return half of the liquid to the pot. Add the chicken, carrots, potatoes, and

tomatoes; bring to a simmer and cook for 1 1/2 hours.

YIELD: Serves 12
SODIUM CONTENT: 105 mg. of sodium per serving

CHICKEN CURRY WITH COCONUT MILK

INGREDIENTS
- 3 boneless, skinless chicken breasts (6 half breasts)
- 1/2 c. all-purpose flour
- freshly ground black pepper to taste
- 5 tbsp. unsalted butter
- 1 medium onion, chopped
- 2 cloves garlic, minced
- 2 green peppers, diced
- 3 tbsp. unsalted curry powder
- 2 c. diced tomatoes
- 2 tbsp. salt-free tomato paste dissolved in 1/4 c. water
- 15-oz. can coconut milk
- 3 tbsp. tamarind paste dissolved in 1/2 c. water and strained
- 1/4 c. dried currants
- 1/4 c. golden raisins

DIRECTIONS:

1. Preheat the oven to 350 degrees. Rinse each piece of chicken breast and pat it dry, then cut it in half to create a total of 12 pieces of chicken. Combine the flour and black pepper and sprinkle over the chicken to coat each piece. Melt 3 tablespoons of the butter in a large skillet on top of the stove and brown the chicken pieces in it, then remove them and set them aside. Add the onion, garlic, and green pepper to the skillet along with the rest of the butter, and cook for several minutes over medium heat, stirring occasionally, until the onions begin to soften and turn brown. Add the curry powder; stir to blend, and cook for 2 minutes.

2. Add the tomatoes, dissolved tomato paste, and coconut milk, and stir to combine. Add the water with dissolved tamarind pulp, making sure you have strained out the skin and seeds (or add the mixture of prune juice and lemon juice if you don't have tamarind paste); stir to blend, then stir in the currants and raisins. Bring this mixture to a simmer, then remove it from the heat.

3. Put the chicken pieces in a large casserole or ovenproof Dutch oven and pour the curry-coconut milk mixture over them, then stir to combine. Cover and bake in the oven until the chicken is tender and the flavors are well developed, about 45 minutes. Allow the mixture to cool

slightly before serving with rice and plain yogurt.

YIELD : Serves 6
SODIUM CONTENT: 34 mg. of sodium per serving

HUNTER'S CHICKEN

- **Ingredients**
- 2 tbsp. olive oil
- 6 chicken drumsticks, washed and excess fat removed
- 6 chicken thighs, washed and excess fat removed
- 1 c. flour
- 3 carrots, chopped
- 3 celery stalks, chopped
- 1 small onion, sliced
- freshly ground black pepper to taste
- 1 tbsp. ground thyme
- 1 tsp. ground sage
- 32-ounce can salt-free whole tomatoes or 3 c. chopped fresh tomatoes
- 1 c. white wine
- 14 shiitake mushrooms, cleaned and sliced
- 2 cloves garlic
- 1 bay leaf

DIRECTIONS:
1. Heat the oil to medium-high heat in a large stew pot or Dutch oven. Roll the chicken in the flour. Add the chicken to the pan and brown well. When the chicken has browned, remove it and add carrots, celery, and onion. Season with black pepper, thyme, and sage. Cook for 10 minutes over medium heat until the vegetables have wilted. Add the chicken, tomatoes, and wine, and stir to combine. Then add mushrooms, garlic, and bay leaf. Bring the mixture to a simmer and cook for 1 1/2 hours. Remove the bay leaf before serving. Serve with rice.

YIELD : Serves 6
SODIUM CONTENT: 147 mg. of sodium per serving

BULGUR STUFFING

INGREDIENTS
- 1/2 c. unsalted butter (one stick)
- 2 large onions, chopped
- 1 1/2 tsp. ground coriander

- 1/2 tsp. ground cumin
- 1 1/2 c. slivered, blanched almonds
- 1 1/2 c. coarsely chopped dried apricots
- 1 1/2 c. raisins
- 4 c. cooked bulgur
- 2 tsp. cinnamon
- 1/2 tsp. ground cloves
- freshly ground pepper to taste

DIRECTIONS:

1. Melt the butter in large skillet. Add the onions, coriander, and cumin. Cover and cook, stirring occasionally, until the onion is translucent, about 10 minutes. Add the almonds, apricots, and raisins. Cook uncovered, stirring occasionally, until the almonds are golden. Transfer to a large bowl. Add the bulgur, cinnamon, cloves, and pepper, and mix well. Refrigerate before using to stuff a turkey before roasting.

YIELD : Serves 8
SODIUM CONTENT: 14 mg. of sodium per serving

CHESTNUT STUFFING

INGREDIENTS

- 1 lb. chestnuts
- 1 tbsp. olive oil
- 1 medium onion, chopped
- 2 tbsp. finely minced fresh sage leaves
- 3/4 lb. ground pork
- freshly ground black pepper to taste
- 2 shallots, finely minced
- 1/2 c. chopped parsley
- 1 tbsp. fresh thyme or 1 tsp. dried thyme
- 2 cloves garlic, minced
- 2 c. salt-free bread crumbs
- 1 bay leaf

DIRECTIONS:

1. Prepare the chestnuts by cutting a cross in the flat side of each one, dropping them into a pot of boiling water, and allowing them to boil for about 5 minutes. Then turn off the heat and remove the chestnuts one by one, peeling off the inner and outer shells. Break the chestnut meats into small pieces with your fingers and put them in a large bowl.

2.   Heat the olive oil in a skillet; add the onion and cook over medium heat, stirring occasionally, until the onion wilts and grows transparent. Add the sage and the bay leaf and cook for a few minutes more. Then add the ground pork and cook, breaking up the pork and stirring it with a heavy spoon so that it browns evenly. When the pork has browned, sprinkle generously with black pepper. Add the pork mixture to the chestnuts and stir to blend. Then add the rest of the ingredients, stir to combine, and sprinkle with a little more black pepper.

YIELD : Serves 8
SODIUM CONTENT: 35 mg. of sodium per serving

JALAPEÑO CORNBREAD STUFFING

INGREDIENTS

- 1 c. milk
- 1 egg
- 1 tbsp. honey
- 1 jalapeño pepper, seeded and finely chopped
- 5 tbsp. unsalted butter
- 1 c. cornmeal
- 1 c. all-purpose flour
- 2 tbsp. low-sodium baking powder
- 2 c. sliced mushrooms
- 2 tsp. sage
- freshly ground black pepper to taste

DIRECTIONS:

1. Preheat the oven to 350 degrees. Lightly grease an 8-inch square baking pan or loaf pan of similar size. Stir together the milk, egg, honey, and chopped pepper in a large bowl until well blended. Melt 3 tablespoons of the butter and add it to the milk mixture. Sift together the cornmeal, flour, and baking powder in a separate bowl and add them to the wet ingredients. Stir only until the dry ingredients are moistened. Pour the batter into the pan and bake for 20 to 25 minutes, until a toothpick dipped into the center of the cornbread comes out clean. Set aside to cool.

2. Melt the remaining butter in a small frying pan. Add the mushrooms and 1 teaspoon of the sage and cook over moderate heat, stirring constantly, for about 3 minutes, or until the mushrooms have begun to soften and absorb the butter. Crumble up the cornbread in a large bowl; add the mushrooms, the remaining sage, and the pepper. Stir until thoroughly blended.

YIELD : Serves 8
SODIUM CONTENT: 26 mg. of sodium per serving

TURKEY BREAST WITH CORNBREAD STUFFING

INGREDIENTS

FOR THE CORNBREAD:

- 1 c. cornmeal
- 1 c. all-purpose flour
- 5 tsp. low-sodium baking powder
- 1 c. milk
- 1 egg
- 3 tbsp. unsalted butter, melted
- 1 tbsp. honey

FOR THE TURKEY AND STUFFING:

- olive oil
- 1 medium onion, chopped
- 1 shallot, chopped
- 1 large clove garlic, minced
- 1 tbsp. chopped fresh sage leaves or 1 tsp. dried sage
- 1 c. sliced mushrooms
- juice of 1/2 lemon
- 1/2 lb. ground pork
- freshly ground black pepper to taste
- 4 tsp. salt-free chili powder
- 1 c. fresh or salt-free frozen corn
- 2 c. crumbled cornbread from this recipe
- 1/4 c. parsley leaves
- 1 bay leaf
- 1 tsp. fresh thyme or 1/2 tsp. dried thyme
- 1 (4-lb.) boneless turkey breast
- 1 c. low-sodium chicken broth

DIRECTIONS:

1. To make the cornbread, preheat the oven to 350 degrees while you sift together the cornmeal, flour, and baking powder in a bowl. Put the milk in a separate bowl; add the egg and beat with a whisk to blend. Then slowly pour in the melted butter, stirring constantly, followed by

the honey. Pour this mixture over the dry ingredients and stir only until the dry ingredients are well moistened. Pour the batter into a lightly greased 8" × 8" baking pan and bake for about 25 minutes until the top just begins to brown and a toothpick inserted into the center of the cornbread comes out clean. Allow to cool. Then crumble up enough of the cornbread to fill 2 cups.

2. To make the stuffing, heat 1 tablespoon of olive oil in a sauté pan. Add the onion, shallot, and garlic, and cook over medium heat, stirring occasionally, until the onion begins to wilt. Add the sage leaves and cook for a few more minutes. Add the mushrooms and cook until they begin to soften. Sprinkle with lemon juice and stir to blend. Then add the ground pork and stir with a wooden spoon until it is evenly browned. Sprinkle with black pepper, add 3 teaspoons of the chili powder, and stir to blend. Transfer this mixture to a large bowl; add 2 cups of crumbled cornbread, corn, parsley, bay leaf, and thyme, and stir to combine.

3. Rinse the turkey breast and pat dry. Spread the meat out flat with the skin side down and "butterfly" the thick part of the breast: Start in the middle of the breast and cut about halfway through the thick section, cutting sideways toward the end, keeping the flat of the knife parallel with the work surface. Fold out the flap of meat created by this cut. Spread stuffing generously across the surface of the meat, using your fingers to press it down tightly. Then roll up the meat around the stuffing to form a cylinder, and use butcher's twine to tie it together. Start with one tie at the middle and add one or two more toward the ends.

4. Wipe the bottom of a roasting pan with olive oil and place the tied turkey breast in it, seam side down. Brush the top of the breast with olive oil and dust lightly with the remaining teaspoon of chili powder. Spread any leftover stuffing around the breast on the bottom of the pan, along with 1/2 cup of the chicken broth. Roast at 350 degrees until the breast meat is cooked through, basting occasionally with the rest of the chicken broth. Cooking time should be about 11/2 hours. Transfer the breast and stuffing to a serving platter and garnish with parsley.

Allow the meat to cool a bit before slicing. To serve, cut slices from the end of the rolled breast so that the meat spirals around a portion of stuffing.

YIELD : Serves 10
SODIUM CONTENT: 103 mg. of sodium per serving

POT ROAST

INGREDIENTS

- 2 tbsp. olive oil
- 3- to 4-lb. rump roast
- 1 onion, quartered
- 1 clove garlic, minced
- 1 green pepper, diced
- 1 large carrot, diced

- 1/4 c. roughly chopped parsley
- 1 bay leaf
- 2 sprigs fresh thyme or 1 tbsp. dried thyme
- freshly ground black pepper to taste
- 1/2 c. red wine
- 13/4 c. salt-free beef broth

DIRECTIONS:

1. Heat the oil in a heavy pot or Dutch oven. Add the meat to the pot and brown well on all sides over medium heat. Remove the meat and add the onion, garlic, green pepper, carrot, parsley, bay leaf, thyme, and black pepper. Cook this mixture for about 10 minutes. When the onion is translucent, add the wine and deglaze the pot by using a wooden spoon to scrape bits of meat off the bottom and sides. Then return the meat to the pot, add the broth, and bring the liquid to a boil. Reduce the heat to a simmer and cook for 3 to 4 hours, covered, turning the meat every 30 minutes, until tender.

YIELD : Serves 8
SODIUM CONTENT: 139 mg. of sodium per serving

BEEF STROGANOFF WITH NOODLES

INGREDIENTS

- 2 tbsp. unsalted butter
- 11/2 lbs. London broil sliced into thin 2- to 3-inch strips
- freshly ground black pepper to taste
- 2 tbsp. balsamic vinegar
- 1 medium onion, chopped
- 1/2 c. dry vermouth or white wine
- 11/2 c. sliced mushrooms
- 1 tsp. basil
- 1 tbsp. flour
- 2 tsp. unsalted Dijon mustard
- 1/2 c. sour cream
- **DIRECTIONS:**

1. Melt the butter in a large frying pan and add the beef. Stir with a wooden spoon until the meat is browned on all sides. Sprinkle the meat with black pepper and balsamic vinegar; continue to cook over moderate heat, stirring, until the meat is cooked through. Remove the meat from the pan to a bowl and set aside. Add the onion to the frying pan and cook, stirring, until translucent, about 5 minutes. Add the vermouth, mushrooms, and basil, and cook,

stirring, until the mushrooms have softened and the liquid is reduced by half. Turn the heat to low; add the flour and mustard, and stir, making sure all the flour is absorbed. Return the beef to the frying pan and stir to combine; then add the sour cream and stir to blend. Serve over noodles cooked without salt.

YIELD : Serves 6
SODIUM CONTENT: 79 mg. of sodium per serving

FLANK STEAK WITH PORTOBELLO MUSHROOMS AND WINE

- **Ingredients**
- 1 flank steak
- freshly ground black pepper to taste
- dash of garlic powder
- 1 c. red wine
- 1 shallot, diced
- 2 portobello mushroom caps, cut into slices 1/4-inch thick
- 1 c. drained salt-free canned tomatoes plus 1/2 c. of juice from the can
- 1 tbsp. dried parsley
- pinch of dried oregano

DIRECTIONS:

1. Preheat the oven to 375 degrees and place a shallow roasting pan or ovenproof dish in the oven to heat up. Season the meat with pepper and garlic powder. Heat a heavy skillet to high heat on top of the stove. Sear the steak in the hot skillet on both sides so that it browns thoroughly and juices are sealed in. Transfer the steak to the pan in the oven to finish cooking (about 10 minutes for medium). Then remove it from the oven and set aside.
2. Meanwhile, use half of the wine to deglaze the skillet and allow it to cook until almost gone. Add the shallot and reduce the heat to low. Add the mushrooms; cook 2 minutes per side, then remove them from the skillet. Add the rest of the wine and allow it to cook until almost evaporated. Add the tomato, parsley, and oregano and cook at a simmer for 10 minutes. Return the mushrooms to the skillet on the stove and cook 1 minute to heat through. Slice the steak on the bias, arrange the slices on a plate with the mushrooms and sauce, and serve.

YIELD : Serves 4
SODIUM CONTENT: 161 mg. of sodium per serving

MARINATED PORK TENDERLOIN

- **Ingredients**

- 1 whole pork tenderloin (about 2 to 3 lbs.)
- 1/4 c. balsamic vinegar
- juice of 1/2 lime
- freshly ground black pepper to taste
- 2 tbsp. chopped parsley
- 1 tsp. paprika
- pinch of crushed red pepper flakes
- 3 tbsp. olive oil
- fresh parsley or rosemary for garnish
- **DIRECTIONS**:

1. Remove the silvery membrane and any visible fat from the meat. Mix together all the other ingredients except the oil and parsley for garnish. Place the meat in a shallow dish and cover with the marinade mixture. Allow to sit for at least an hour (the longer it marinates, the better it will be); put it in the refrigerator if you are going to marinate it for several hours.

2. Preheat the oven to 375 degrees. Heat the oil in a heavy ovenproof skillet. When the oil begins to smoke, add the meat and sear it on all sides. Searing each side could take a few minutes. Then place the skillet in the oven and roast for 25 to 30 minutes until it is cooked through (no pink shows when you slice into the middle). To serve, slice the meat at an angle and arrange on a platter, garnished with fresh parsley or rosemary.

YIELD : Serves 6
SODIUM CONTENT: 112 mg. of sodium per serving

SPICY PORK TENDERLOIN

INGREDIENTS

- 1 whole pork tenderloin (2 to 3 lbs.)
- 1 tsp. salt-free chili powder, or more if desired
- 2 tsp. ground cumin
- 1 tsp. powdered ginger
- 1/4 tsp. ground allspice
- 1/4 tsp. paprika
- freshly ground black pepper to taste
- fresh lime wedges

DIRECTIONS:

1. Preheat broiler or prepare the charcoal gill. Wash and dry the pork tenderloin. Combine the spices in a bowl and spread them generously on the surface of the meat so that it is completely coated. Place the meat under the broiler, 4 inches from the heat source, or on the

grill, and cook until the side nearest the heat has browned. Then turn it over and cook for another 15 minutes or so, depending on the thickness of the meat, until it is cooked through. The spices will form a crust. Serve with wedges of fresh lime.

YIELD : Serves 6
SODIUM CONTENT: 112 mg. of sodium per serving

PORK TENDERLOIN WITH MUSHROOM AND HERB SAUCE

- **Ingredients**
- 1 whole pork tenderloin (2 to 3 lbs.)
- freshly ground black pepper to taste
- 1 thin slice unsalted butter (about 1 tsp.)
- 10 white button or other mushrooms
- 2 tbsp. flour
- 1 1/2 c. low-sodium chicken broth
- 1/2 c. heavy cream
- 1 tbsp. fresh lemon juice
- 1 tbsp. chopped fresh parsley
- 1 tbsp. chopped fresh basil
- 2 sage leaves, finely chopped
- 1 tbsp. olive oil

DIRECTIONS:

1. Preheat the oven to 400 degrees. Wash the pork tenderloin, pat dry, trim any excess fat, and sprinkle with black pepper. Heat oil to medium-high in an ovenproof pan. Sear the meat on all sides in the oil, then place in the oven to cook for at least 20 minutes.

2. In the meantime, prepare the sauce. Heat a saucepan to medium-high on top of the stove and add the butter and mushrooms. When they release their liquid, add the flour and cook for 5 minutes more, stirring to make sure the flour doesn't burn. Add the chicken broth and cream, whisk in the lemon juice, and bring to a boil. Lower the heat and simmer until the sauce is reduced by half, then add the herbs and continue to cook 5 minutes or more until the sauce thickens. Reduce the heat to just enough to keep the sauce warm.

3. When the meat has cooked through, remove from the pan and allow to stand for 5 minutes. To serve, slice the meat into thin rounds and arrange them on a plate, then smother them with the sauce.

YIELD : Serves 6
SODIUM CONTENT: 124 mg. of sodium per serving

PORK VINDALOO

INGREDIENTS

- 1 1/2-lb. boneless pork loin, cut into 1-inch cubes
- vegetable oil
- freshly ground black pepper to taste
- 2 c. finely chopped onion
- 1 tbsp. plus 2 tsp. minced garlic
- 1 tbsp. plus 2 tsp. peeled, minced fresh ginger
- 1 1/2 tsp. cumin seeds
- 1 1/2 tsp. mustard seeds
- 4 whole cloves
- 2 1/2 tsp. cayenne pepper
- 1 1/2 tsp. paprika
- 1 1/2 tsp. turmeric
- 1 tsp. ground cinnamon
- 1 c. low-sodium chicken broth
- 2 tbsp. prune juice
- 1 tbsp. lemon juice
- 1 tbsp. cider vinegar
- 1 tbsp. molasses
- chopped cilantro leaves for garnish

DIRECTIONS:

1. If the pork is moist, pat it dry with paper towels. Heat a small amount of vegetable oil in a large pot or Dutch oven and brown the cubes of meat on all sides. Sprinkle the meat with black pepper and stir to distribute.

2. Remove the meat from the pot and set it aside. Add another tablespoon or two of oil to the pot; add the onion and cook over moderate heat, stirring frequently, for several minutes until it is well browned. Add the garlic and ginger; stir and continue to cook. Grind up the cumin, mustard seeds, and cloves, and mix them with the cayenne pepper, paprika, turmeric, and cinnamon. Add the spice mixture to the pot and continue to cook for a minute, stirring. Then return the browned meat to the pot and stir to combine.

3. Pour the chicken broth, prune juice, lemon juice, vinegar, and molasses over the mixture in the pot. Bring to a simmer; cover and continue to simmer over low heat for an hour, until the flavors are well blended and the meat is fork tender. If oil rises to the top, skim it off with a spoon. If the vindaloo seems too thin, turn up the heat and allow the sauce to cook down.

Transfer to a serving dish and sprinkle fresh cilantro leaves across the top before serving.

YIELD: Serves 6
SODIUM CONTENT: 83 mg. of sodium per serving

TUSCAN-STYLE BRAISED PORK LOIN

- **Ingredients**
- olive oil
- 1 large pork loin (3 to 4 lbs.)
- 3 carrots, peeled and chopped
- 2 stalks celery, chopped
- 1 onion, diced
- 1 bunch fresh thyme
- 2 sticks fresh rosemary
- 1/2 c. chopped parsley
- 28-oz. can unsalted tomatoes or about 2 c. fresh tomatoes
- 1 c. white wine
- 2 (15-oz.) cans salt-free navy beans or 4 c. dry beans, cooked

DIRECTIONS:

1. Heat a small amount of oil to high in a large ovenproof pot or Dutch oven on top of the stove. Add the meat and sear on all sides. Remove the meat and add the carrots, celery, onion, black pepper, and herbs. Reduce the heat to medium and cook for 10 minutes, stirring occasionally to prevent burning
2. Preheat the oven to 325 degrees. Add the tomatoes and wine to the pot, then stir and scrape the bottom and sides of the pan to deglaze. Drain the beans and add them to the pot, then return the pork to the pot, cover, and cook in the oven for about 2 1/2 hours, until the pork is very tender.

YIELD: Serves 8
SODIUM CONTENT: 165 mg. of sodium per serving

GREEN CHILI STEW

INGREDIENTS

- olive oil
- 2 1/2- to 3-lb. top round pork roast
- freshly ground black pepper to taste
- 1 medium onion, diced
- 6 long green chilies, diced

- 12 c. water
- 1 c. red wine
- 1 tsp. dried thyme or 2 tsp. fresh thyme leaves
- 1/4 c. finely chopped parsley
- 4 large potatoes, peeled and diced

DIRECTIONS:

1. In a large stew pot or Dutch oven, heat a little oil to medium-high heat on top of the stove. Season the meat with pepper, add it to the pot, and brown it on all sides. Remove the meat; add the onion and chiles, and cook for 10 minutes, stirring occasionally. Return the roast to the pot and add the water, wine, thyme, and parsley. Cover the stew and simmer for 2 hours.
2. Add the potatoes and cook for another 1/2 hour. Remove the roast from the pot and use a fork to pull it apart, shredding the meat. Return the meat to the pot and continue to cook until it is heated through. Serve with crusty salt-free bread.

YIELD : Serves 8
SODIUM CONTENT: 109 mg. of sodium per serving

BRAISED PORK CHOPS WITH PORTOBELLO MUSHROOMS

- **Ingredients**
- 1 tbsp. olive oil
- 2 thick boneless pork chops
- 2 portobello mushrooms, sliced into strips 1/4-inch thick
- freshly ground black pepper to taste
- 2 cloves garlic, diced
- 1 tbsp. unsalted tomato paste
- 1/2 c. low-sodium chicken broth

DIRECTIONS:

1. Heat the oil in a sauté pan and add the chops. Brown well on both sides, then remove to a plate. Add the mushrooms and black pepper and cook 5 minutes, then add the garlic and cook 2 minutes longer. Add the tomato paste and chicken broth, and stir together. Return the chops to the pan, and cook covered for 10 minutes, then remove the cover and cook for 5 minutes more, or until the chops are cooked through.

YIELD : Serves 2
SODIUM CONTENT: 104 mg. of sodium per serving

PORK CHOPS WITH TOMATOES AND

PEPPERS

- **Ingredients**
- 2 tbsp. olive oil
- 5 center-cut pork chops
- 1 c. white wine
- 2 cloves garlic, minced
- 1 medium onion, chopped
- 1 medium green pepper, roughly chopped
- 2 medium tomatoes, chopped, or 2 c. salt-free canned tomatoes
- 1 tbsp. fresh basil or 2 tsp. dried basil
- 1 sprig of fresh thyme or 1 tsp. dried thyme
- 2 tbsp. balsamic vinegar

DIRECTIONS:

1. Heat the oil in a skillet large enough to hold all the pork chops. Brown the chops on both sides and remove to a plate. Pour 1/4 cup of white wine into the pan and stir with a wooden spoon to deglaze (dissolve the residue of the meat in the wine to create a dark sauce). Add the garlic and onions and cook for several minutes, stirring, until the onions become translucent. Add the green pepper and cook for another minute or so, until it begins to soften. Add the tomatoes, basil, thyme, vinegar, and the rest of the wine. Allow the mixture to cook for about 2 minutes over medium heat so that the flavors begin to combine

2. Return the pork chops to the pan, including any juice that has drained off them while they were out of the pan. Distribute the chops so that all are at least partially covered by the sauce. Bring the mixture to a boil, then reduce the heat to low; cover and simmer for about 40 minutes, until the pork chops are thoroughly cooked and tender. If the mixture seems too liquid after 30 minutes, remove the cover so that the sauce cooks down for the last several minutes. Serve with rice.

YIELD : Serves 5
SODIUM CONTENT: 80 mg. of sodium per serving

PORK CHOPS WITH APPLES

INGREDIENTS

- 2 tbsp. vegetable oil
- 1 tbsp. unsalted butter
- 6 center-cut pork chops
- 3/4 c. white wine
- 4 apples, peeled, cored, and cut into eight sections each

- ground cumin
- freshly ground black pepper to taste
- 2 tbsp. calvados (optional)

DIRECTIONS:

1. Preheat the oven to 350 degrees. Heat the oil in a large iron skillet, then melt the butter in it and stir to blend. Remove any excess fat from the pork chops. Brown them in the skillet on both sides, then remove. Add 1/4 cup of the white wine and deglaze (stir to scrape bits of meat off the bottom and sides of the pan). Then add the pieces of apple, spreading them evenly in the pan. Rub a small amount of cumin on both sides of each pork chop, then return the chops to the pan, arranging them on top of the apples
2. Sprinkle them with black pepper and pour the rest of the wine over them, followed by the calvados. Put the pan on the middle rack of the oven and cook for about 40 minutes, until the pork chops are cooked through. Serve each chop smothered in apples.

YIELD : Serves 6
SODIUM CONTENT: 73 mg. of sodium per serving

STUFFED PORK CHOPS

- **Ingredients**
- 1 tbsp. unsalted butter
- 1 shallot, minced
- freshly ground black pepper to taste
- 10 mushrooms, sliced (use cremini or porcini, if you can find them—otherwise use supermarket button mushrooms)
- 1/4 c. low-sodium chicken broth
- 2 tbsp. finely chopped parsley
- 1 tsp. chopped rosemary
- 4 thick pork chops
- olive oil

DIRECTIONS:

1. Heat a skillet; add butter and shallot, and cook for 5 minutes over medium heat. Add the mushrooms and black pepper and allow the mushrooms to cook down for about 10 minutes, reducing the heat if necessary to prevent burning. Add the broth and deglaze the pan by stirring to dissolve cooked bits of vegetables clinging to the pan. Add parsley and rosemary; turn up the heat and reduce the liquid until the pan is almost dry. Remove this mushroom mixture to a plate and allow it to cool.
2. Preheat the oven to 350 degrees. Wash the pork chops and pat them dry. Use a sharp knife to cut sideways into each chop to create a pocket. Fill the pockets with the mushroom mixture.

Heat a small amount of olive oil in the skillet and sear the chops on both sides. Transfer the chops to a baking dish, put them in the oven, and bake until cooked through, 20 to 30 minutes.

YIELD : Serves 4
SODIUM CONTENT: 80 mg. of sodium per serving

MELISSA FLOOD' S PULLED PORK

INGREDIENTS
FOR THE RUB:
- 2 tbsp. sugar
- 2 tbsp. brown sugar
- 2 tbsp. ground cumin
- 2 tbsp. salt-free chili powder
- 2 tbsp. freshly ground black pepper
- 1 tbsp. cayenne pepper
- 1/4 c. Hungarian paprika

FOR THE PORK:
- 1 large boned pork loin (6 to 8 lbs.)
- 2/3 c. orange juice
- 2/3 c. molasses
- 1/3 c. cider vinegar or balsamic vinegar

DIRECTIONS:
1. Mix the spices for the rub together and spread them generously over the surface of the pork loin. Put the excess in a jar to save for future use. Allow the rubbed pork to sit for 2 hours.
2. Preheat the oven to 200 degrees. Put the pork in a roasting pan, cover it with aluminum foil, and roast it in the oven at this low heat until a meat thermometer inserted in the middle of the loin reaches 170 degrees. This could take a few hours.
3. Remove the loin from the oven, allow it to cool, and shred it into bite-sized pieces with your fingers. Return this "pulled" pork to the pan, and add 1/2 cup of water. Mix the orange juice, molasses, and vinegar, and pour the mixture over the pulled pork.
4. Return the pork to the 200-degree oven and cook for another hour.
5. Taste the pork; if it seems too dry, add a bit of water and cook a bit more; if it seems too spicy, add a little molasses and orange juice. Serve it warm.

YIELD : Serves 20
SODIUM CONTENT: 103 mg. of sodium per serving

RIBS

INGREDIENTS
- 2 racks baby back pork spareribs (1 lb. each), cut in half
- 1 onion
- 6 c. Andersons' Famous Barbecue Sauce
- **DIRECTIONS**:

1. Bring a large pot of water to a boil on top of the stove, reduce the heat to a simmer, and add the ribs and onion. Simmer for 45 minutes, then remove the ribs and let them rest for 30 minutes (if you wish, you can simmer the ribs the day before and keep them in the refrigerator until ready to use).
2. Preheat the oven to 250 degrees. Add the ribs to a shallow roasting pan and cover with half the sauce. Put them in the oven and roast for 1 1/2 hours, basting every 30 minutes with the rest of the sauce. The longer you cook them at low heat, the better they will be (we have cooked them for as long as 4 hours). If you are going to cook the ribs outdoors on a charcoal or gas grill, make sure that the heat is very low. Place the ribs on the grill and baste with sauce, turning frequently (every 10 minutes) for 40 minutes or longer.

YIELD : Serves 4
SODIUM CONTENT: 175 mg. of sodium per serving

VEAL CHOPS WITH MUSHROOMS AND PARSLEY

- **Ingredients**
- 2 tbsp. olive oil
- 4 veal chops
- 1 shallot or 1/2 medium onion, chopped
- 1/2 c. white wine or dry vermouth
- 2 c. sliced mushrooms (cremini or porcini, if you can find them—otherwise use supermarket button mushrooms)
- juice of 1/2 lemon
- freshly ground black pepper to taste
- 1/2 c. chopped Italian parsley
- 2 sprigs fresh thyme or 2 tsp. dried thyme

DIRECTIONS:

1. Heat the oil in a frying pan large enough to hold all the chops; brown the chops on both sides. Remove them from the pan and set them aside. Add the chopped shallot or onion to the pan

and cook for several minutes until it turns translucent. Add 2 tablespoons of the wine to the pan and deglaze it by stirring with a wooden spoon so that the residue from browning the meat dissolves in the liquid. Add the mushrooms and allow them to cook, stirring occasionally, for about 5 minutes, until they begin to soften. Sprinkle the mushrooms with lemon juice and black pepper. Add parsley and thyme; stir them into the mushroom mixture and cook for another 3 to 5 minutes, until all the parsley wilts.

2. Return the chops and the juice that has drained off them to the pan and distribute them on top of the mushrooms. Add the rest of the wine, bring to a boil, then reduce the heat to low. Cover and simmer until the chops are cooked through, about 25 minutes. To serve, put a chop on a plate and cover it with a generous spoonful of mushrooms and sauce.

YIELD: Serves 4
SODIUM CONTENT: 160 mg. of sodium per serving

VEAL CHOPS WITH RED PEPPER SAUCE

- **Ingredients**
- 3 sweet red peppers
- olive oil
- 4 veal chops or medallions
- freshly ground black pepper to taste
- 1 shallot, minced
- 1/4 c. white wine
- 2 tbsp. dry vermouth
- 1 1/2 c. heavy cream
- 1 tbsp. finely chopped parsley

DIRECTIONS:

1. Heat the oven to 350 degrees. Place the whole red peppers on a baking sheet, brush them with olive oil, and roast them on the middle rack of the oven until tender, about 1/2 hour.

2. In the meantime, rinse the meat and pat dry with a paper towel. Sprinkle both sides with black pepper and rub the pepper into the surface of the meat. Heat a small amount of oil over medium-high heat in a skillet, and sear the meat on both sides. Transfer the meat to a shallow pan and place it in the oven to finish cooking. This should take 15 to 20 minutes, depending on the thickness of the chops or medallions.

3. When the peppers are cooked, remove them from the oven, cut off the tops, and remove the seeds and pulp; use a blender or food processor to reduce them to a smooth purée. Then heat 2 tablespoons of oil in a saucepan; add the shallot and cook over medium heat for 3 or 4 minutes, until transparent. Be careful not to burn the shallot. Add the wine, vermouth, and

heavy cream. Reduce the heat so the cream comes to a simmer without rising over the edges of the pot. When the cream has reduced by half, add the pepper purée and parsley, and stir to combine well. Sprinkle with black pepper.

4. Keep the sauce warm on very low heat until the veal has cooked. To serve, ladle a generous portion of sauce over each veal chop or medallion.

YIELD : Serves 4

SODIUM CONTENT: 154 mg. of sodium per serving

VEAL CHOPS WITH SOUR CHERRY AND PORT WINE SAUCE

- **Ingredients**
- 1 tbsp. unsalted butter
- 1 small shallot, minced
- 1 c. dried sour cherries
- 3 sage leaves, torn in half
- 1 c. port wine
- 1/4 c. low-sodium chicken broth
- 1 tbsp. olive oil
- freshly ground black pepper to taste
- 4 veal chops

DIRECTIONS:

1. To make the sauce, heat the butter in a saucepan, add the shallot, and sauté for 6 minutes. Add the cherries and sage and cook for another 5 minutes. Then add port wine and chicken broth, and cook at a simmer for 15 minutes. When it has cooked, strain the sauce and keep warm.

2. To cook the chops, preheat the oven to 400 degrees. Heat the oil in a sauté pan over medium-high heat, season the chops with black pepper, and add them to the pan, browning them well on both sides. Transfer the chops to a shallow roasting pan and put them in the oven until cooked through, about 12 to 15 minutes, depending on the thickness of the chops. Serve the sauce over the chops.

YIELD : Serves 4

SODIUM CONTENT: 176 mg. of sodium per serving

BRAISED DOUBLE THICK VEAL CHOPS

- **Ingredients**

- 4 large tomatoes, or enough to make 3 1/2 to 4 c. of purée
- 1/2 c. heavy cream
- 1 shallot, peeled and quartered
- 3 cloves garlic
- 1/4 c. roughly chopped parsley
- freshly ground black pepper to taste
- 1/4 tsp. ground thyme
- 1 tbsp. balsamic vinegar
- olive oil
- 4 veal chops, about 1 1/2-to 2-inch thick

DIRECTIONS:
1. Quarter and seed the tomatoes; put them in a blender or food processor and blend until liquefied. Add all the rest of the ingredients except the veal chops and olive oil, and blend until smooth. Place this mixture in a pan and cook over medium-low heat until reduced by one-third. Cover and set aside.
2. In a pan large enough to hold all the ingredients, bring a small amount of oil to high heat and sear the chops so that they are well browned on all sides. Add the sauce and turn the chops so that they are evenly coated with it. Cover the pot and simmer until the veal is very tender, about an hour or more. Serve hot.

YIELD : Serves 4
SODIUM CONTENT: 216 mg. of sodium per serving

ROASTED VEAL WITH SHALLOTS

INGREDIENTS
- 2 tbsp. olive oil
- freshly ground black pepper to taste
- 4-lb. veal roast, rolled and tied
- 10 to 12 shallots, peeled and sliced
- 1 c. white wine
- 1/2 c. low-sodium chicken broth
- 3 cloves garlic, peeled and left whole
- 2 fresh bay leaves
- 3 tbsp. chopped parsley

DIRECTIONS:
1. Heat the oil over medium-high heat in a large pot. Rub pepper into the surface of the roast; sear the roast on all sides, and remove it to a plate. Add the shallots; reduce the heat to

medium-low and cook for 8 to 10 minutes. Add the wine and use a wooden spoon to deglaze the pot, scraping up the bits of meat that cling to the bottom. Add the broth, garlic, bay leaves, and parsley and return the meat to the pot. Cover and simmer at a gentle, low heat for 2 1/2 to 3 hours, turning the roast from time to time so it cooks evenly.

YIELD : Serves 8
SODIUM CONTENT: 164 mg. of sodium per serving

BRAISED VEAL LOIN WITH SAGE AND PEARS

INGREDIENTS

- 3 tbsp. olive oil
- 3 1/2- to 4-lb. veal loin
- freshly ground black pepper to taste
- 1 medium onion, diced
- 2 celery stalks, diced
- 3 carrots, diced
- 8 fresh sage leaves
- 1 c. low-sodium chicken broth
- 1 c. water
- 1/4 c. chopped parsley
- 5 Seckel pears, quartered and pitted, or 3 larger pears, quartered and pitted
- **DIRECTIONS**:

1. Preheat the oven to 325 degrees. Heat 3 tablespoons of olive oil over high heat on the top of the stove in a large Dutch oven or other ovenproof pot. Season the veal loin with pepper and sear it on all sides in the oil. Remove the veal from the pot, set aside, and add the onion, celery, and carrots. Reduce heat to medium. After 5 minutes, season with pepper. Add sage leaves and cook for another 10 minutes, stirring occasionally to prevent burning. Add broth and water, and stir to deglaze the pot, scraping up the bits of meat and vegetables that cling to the bottom and sides. Add the parsley and pears, and return the veal loin to the pot. Cover and place in the oven; cook for 2 to 2 1/2 hours or until the meat is very tender.

YIELD : Serves 8
SODIUM CONTENT: 168 mg. of sodium per serving

OSSO BUCO

INGREDIENTS

- 4 veal shanks with bones, 1 1/2 inches thick (with marrow)

- flour
- 2 tbsp. high-quality olive oil
- 1 c. finely chopped onion
- 2/3 c. finely chopped carrots
- 2/3 c. finely chopped green pepper
- 2 tsp. finely chopped garlic
- 1 c. dry white wine
- 1 c. low-sodium beef broth or water
- 1 1/2 c. canned salt-free tomatoes or 2 medium fresh tomatoes
- 1 sprig fresh thyme
- 2 bay leaves
- 3 sprigs finely chopped parsley
- freshly ground black pepper to taste

DIRECTIONS:

1. Preheat the oven to 350 degrees. Use butcher's twine to tie the meat around the bone so that it holds together while it cooks. Put some flour on a plate, and dredge the meat in the flour. Heat the oil on medium-high in a heavy bottomed pot large enough to hold all the pieces of meat without overlapping. When the oil begins to smoke, add the veal shanks and brown them quickly on all sides; remove the shanks from the pot. Add the onion, carrots, and green pepper to the pot and sauté for 6 to 8 minutes, until the onion becomes translucent and the vegetables release their flavor. Watch the heat to make sure the vegetables don't burn. Add the garlic and cook another 3 minutes. Then add the wine to deglaze the pot, scraping up bits of meat and vegetables from the bottom and sides, and cook down for 4 minutes.
2. Return the veal shanks to the pot; add the rest of the ingredients and bring to a simmer. Then place the pot, tightly covered, in the oven and cook for 4 hours. Baste and turn the meat at least every half hour. Remove thyme and bay leaves before serving.

YIELD: Serves 6
SODIUM CONTENT: 168 mg. of sodium per serving

VEAL SCALOPPINE

INGREDIENTS

- 1/2 c. flour
- 1 tsp. salt-free chili powder
- freshly ground black pepper to taste
- 8 to 12 veal scaloppine slices (about 1 lb.), pounded to 1/4-inch thick
- 2 tbsp. olive oil

- 2 tbsp. unsalted butter
- juice of 1 lemon

DIRECTIONS:

1. Spread the flour on a plate; add the chili powder and a generous grinding of pepper, and stir to combine. Dredge the slices of meat in the flour mixture so they are lightly coated. Heat a sauté pan or skillet over medium-high heat, then add 1 tablespoon of the olive oil and 1 tablespoon of the unsalted butter. When the butter has melted, stir to combine it with the oil. Add the meat slices to the pan two or three at a time, and cook a minute or so on each side so that they just cook through. Add small amounts of oil and butter if the pan begins to dry out. As they cook, transfer the meat slices to a baking dish and sprinkle with lemon juice and a light grinding of pepper. Put the baking dish in a 250-degree oven to stay warm while you finish cooking the meat. Serve immediately.

YIELD: Serves 8
SODIUM CONTENT: 88 mg. of sodium per serving

IRISH LAMB STEW

- **Ingredients**
- 2 lbs. lamb shoulder cut into 1-inch cubes
- 2 tbsp. flour
- freshly ground black pepper to taste
- 1 tbsp. vegetable oil
- 1 c. boiling water
- 1 c. white wine
- 1 bay leaf
- 1 c. sliced carrots (1/2-inch slices)
- 1 c. cubed turnip (1/2-inch cubes)
- 1 c. peeled, cubed potato (1/2-inch cubes)
- 1 medium onion, sliced
- 2 tbsp. cider vinegar
- 2 tsp. fresh thyme or 1 tsp. dried thyme
- parsley or fresh thyme for garnish

DIRECTIONS:

1. Trim the fat off the cubes of meat and sprinkle them with flour and ground pepper. Heat oil in a heavy pot or Dutch oven; add the meat and turn the pieces until they are browned on all sides. Pour boiling water over the meat (watch out for splattering when the water hits the oil), then add wine and bay leaf. Simmer, covered, over low heat for an hour or until the meat

becomes fork-tender. Stir occasionally to prevent the meat from sticking and burning on the bottom.

2. Add the vegetables, sprinkle with cider vinegar, thyme, and a grinding of fresh pepper, and stir to combine. Simmer another 1/2 hour, until the vegetables are cooked through. If the stew seems dry, add a little more water or white wine. Remove the bay leaf and serve garnished with parsley or a sprig of thyme.

YIELD: Serves 6
SODIUM CONTENT: 108 mg. of sodium per serving

SHISH KEBABS

INGREDIENTS
FOR THE KEBABS:
- 1 1/2 lbs. lamb, cut into 1-inch cubes
- several bay leaves
- 2 green peppers, diced in large pieces
- 1 large onion, diced in large pieces
- 2 pints cherry tomatoes
- 2 pints mushrooms, stalks removed

FOR THE MARINADE:
- 1/2 c. balsamic vinegar
- 1/2 c. olive oil
- 2 tbsp. salt-free Dijon mustard
- 2 cloves garlic, minced
- freshly ground black pepper to taste

DIRECTIONS:
1. Place the cubes of meat in a shallow bowl. Whisk together the marinade ingredients, pour them over the meat, and stir to make sure all the cubes are covered in the liquid. Put in the refrigerator to marinate for 2 to 3 hours.
2. Prepare the charcoal grill: light the charcoal, and allow it to burn down until the coals turn gray and glow evenly. Put the meat on one set of skewers, interspersing pieces of bay leaf between cubes of meat. Put the vegetables on another set of skewers in order to cook them separately. Prepare the vegetable skewers by alternating tomatoes, mushroom caps, pieces of pepper, and onion. Place the meat skewers on the hottest part of the fire and the vegetable skewers on a cooler part. Cook, turning frequently to prevent burning, until meat and vegetables are cooked through. Serve immediately with rice.

YIELD: 6 kebabs
SODIUM CONTENT: 107 mg. of sodium per kebab

MEATBALLS

INGREDIENTS

- 2 lbs. ground beef
- 1/4 c. finely chopped parsley
- 6 cloves garlic, minced fine
- freshly ground black pepper to taste
- 2 tbsp. finely chopped basil
- 1 egg
- 1/2 c. salt-free bread crumbs
- olive oil

DIRECTIONS:

1. Place all the ingredients except the bread crumbs and oil in a bowl and use your fingers to mix them together, squeezing the other ingredients through the ground meat. Add bread crumbs sparingly in order to reduce the moisture in the mixture and tighten it up. Take small pieces of meat and form them into balls about 1 1/2 inches in diameter by rolling them between your palms. Continue until all the meat is used up. Put the meatballs on a plate and set aside to rest for at least 15 minutes before cooking.
2. Heat a small amount of oil over medium-high heat in a nonstick frying pan. Cook a few meatballs at a time so as not to crowd the pan. Turn the meatballs as they cook to sear them on all sides. Leave them in the pan until cooked through; we like them best if still a little pink inside.

YIELD: 18 meatballs
SODIUM CONTENT: 115 mg. of sodium per 3-meatball serving

GREEN PEPPERS STUFFED WITH MEAT AND RICE

INGREDIENTS

- 4 medium green peppers
- olive oil
- 1 medium onion, chopped
- 1 c. sliced mushrooms
- 1 tbsp. lemon juice
- 3/4 lb. ground beef (at least 70 percent lean)
- 1 tbsp. balsamic vinegar
- freshly ground black pepper to taste

- 1 tbsp. unsalted tomato paste
- 1 tbsp. fresh unsalted horseradish
- 1 tsp. fresh thyme or 1/2 tsp. dried thyme
- 1 c. cooked brown or white rice
- 1/4 c. salt-free bread crumbs (optional,)

DIRECTIONS:

1. Preheat the oven to 350 degrees. Cut the tops off the peppers and remove the pulp and seeds to create shells. Place them cut side down on a baking sheet and brush the outsides lightly with olive oil. Put in the oven and bake for about 20 minutes, until the shells are tender but firm enough to hold their shape.
2. Meanwhile, heat 2 tablespoons olive oil in a large skillet, add the onion, and cook for several minutes, until translucent. Add the mushrooms and cook for about 5 minutes, until they begin to soften. Sprinkle with lemon juice. Add the meat and push it around with a wooden spoon until it is thoroughly browned. Sprinkle the meat with balsamic vinegar and ground pepper. Add the tomato paste, horseradish, and thyme, and stir to blend. Cook over moderate heat for about 5 minutes, stirring occasionally to prevent burning.
3. Add the rice to the meat mixture and stir to blend. Spoon the meat and rice into the pepper shells, filling them completely. If you wish, you can sprinkle the top of each one with salt-free bread crumbs. Place the stuffed peppers in a baking dish and return them to the oven for 15 minutes. Serve with a side dish of more rice.

YIELD : Serves 4
SODIUM CONTENT: 40 mg. of sodium per serving

MEATLOAF

INGREDIENTS
- 2 lbs. lean ground beef
- 1/4 c. finely chopped parsley
- 5 basil leaves, finely chopped
- 1 large onion, finely chopped
- 1/4 c. salt-free bread crumbs
- 1 egg
- 1/4 c. salt-free tomato purée
- 1 tbsp. Andersons' Steak Sauce (optional—)
- 1 tbsp. salt-free horseradish (optional—)
- a few drops salt-free hot sauce

DIRECTIONS:

1. Preheat the oven to 375 degrees. Put all the ingredients in a large bowl and squeeze together with your hands until thoroughly combined. If the mixture seems too moist, increase the bread crumbs. Press the meat mixture into a nonstick loaf pan and bake for 1 hour.

YIELD : Serves 8
SODIUM CONTENT: 103 mg. of sodium per serving

SOUTHWEST-STYLE RICE

- **Ingredients**
- 1 tbsp. olive oil
- 1 medium onion, chopped
- 1 clove garlic, minced
- 1 medium yellow or red sweet pepper, cut into 1/2-inch pieces
- 1 lb. lean ground beef
- freshly ground black pepper to taste
- 28-oz. can peeled unsalted tomatoes
- 1 bay leaf
- 1 1/2 c. white or brown rice

DIRECTIONS:

1. Heat the oil in a large, deep skillet or saucepan over a medium flame; add the onion, garlic, and green pepper, and cook for several minutes until the onion becomes translucent. Add the ground beef and stir it around with a wooden spoon until it has browned evenly. Sprinkle black pepper over the meat and stir to blend. Add tomatoes, bay leaf, and rice. Bring to a boil, then reduce the heat and simmer, covered, until the rice has absorbed all the moisture and is well cooked—about 1/2 hour. Remove the bay leaf before serving. This is a great dish to serve with bread or black beans and a touch of Mr. Spice Tangy Bang hot sauce on the side.

YIELD : Serves 4
SODIUM CONTENT: 51 mg. of sodium per serving

SHEPHERD'S PIE

- **Ingredients**
- 2 lbs. Yukon Gold potatoes
- 1/2 c. milk
- 1 1/2 lbs. ground sirloin
- 2 tbsp. balsamic vinegar
- freshly ground black pepper to taste

- 2 tbsp. olive oil
- 1 medium onion, chopped
- 2 c. sliced mushrooms
- 1 medium tomato, chopped
- 1 tsp. thyme, fresh or dried
- juice of 1/2 lemon
- 1 c. roughly chopped parsley
- unsalted butter

DIRECTIONS:

1. Peel and boil the potatoes until they are tender. Mash them, adding the milk, until smooth, and set aside. Brown the meat in a heavy frying pan, stirring with a wooden spoon so that it cooks evenly. Add vinegar and ground pepper and stir to blend. In a separate pan, heat the olive oil and add the onion. Cook for several minutes until the onion turns translucent. Add the mushrooms, tomato, and thyme, and continue to cook until the mushrooms begin to soften. Sprinkle the mixture with lemon juice and black pepper, and stir to blend.

2. Preheat the oven to 350 degrees. Transfer the mushroom mixture to the meat; add the chopped parsley and stir to distribute evenly. Cover and cook over medium heat for 5 minutes. Transfer this mixture to an ovenproof dish. Spread the mashed potatoes on top to form a crust. Dot the potatoes with butter. Bake for 20 minutes. Then turn the heat up to broil for 5 minutes, or until the potatoes are nicely browned.

YIELD: Serves 8
SODIUM CONTENT: 77 mg. of sodium per serving

MOUSSAKA

INGREDIENTS

FOR THE MEAT FILLING:

- 1 tbsp. olive oil
- 2 c. chopped onion
- 3 cloves garlic, finely minced
- 1/2 green pepper, finely chopped
- 1 lb. ground lamb
- 1 lb. ground sirloin
- freshly ground black pepper to taste
- 2 c. chopped tomatoes
- 3 tbsp. unsalted tomato paste
- 3/4 c. red wine

- 2 tbsp. balsamic vinegar
- 2 c. sliced mushrooms
- 1/2 c. fresh chopped parsley
- 1 tsp. thyme
- 1 tsp. cinnamon
- 2 tbsp. lemon juice

FOR THE EGGPLANT:
- 2 medium eggplants
- 1 tbsp. olive oil

FOR THE WHITE SAUCE:
- 1/2 c. flour
- 1/4 tsp. nutmeg
- 1/2 c. unsalted butter, melted
- 4 c. milk
- 2 eggs
- 1/2 c. grated low-sodium Gouda or other low-sodium cheese
-

1. Heat the oil in a large skillet. Add the onions, garlic, and green pepper and cook for several minutes until the onions are translucent. Add the ground meat and cook, stirring with a wooden spoon, until browned. Sprinkle with black pepper; add the tomatoes and tomato paste, and stir to blend. Add the red wine and balsamic vinegar and stir; then add the mushrooms, parsley, thyme, cinnamon, and lemon juice, and stir to blend. Reduce the heat and simmer for 45 minutes.
2. Preheat the oven to 350 degrees. Cut the eggplant into slices 1/2-inch thick. Brush the olive oil on a baking sheet and spread the eggplant slices on it; brush a bit more olive oil on top of the eggplant. Be sure to use the olive oil sparingly. Cover the baking sheet loosely with aluminum foil. Bake for 30 minutes, until the eggplant is tender.
3. To make the white sauce, stir the flour and nutmeg together in a bowl. Add the melted butter to the flour mixture; stir to combine. Place the mixture in the top of a double boiler over boiling water. Bring the milk almost to a boil in a separate pan, then add to the flour-butter mixture. Cook in the double boiler, stirring constantly, until the mixture begins to thicken. Remove from the heat and allow to cool for a few minutes. Beat the eggs in a bowl. Add half of the flour-butter mixture to the bowl, stirring constantly to prevent the eggs from scrambling. When the mixture is uniform, pour it back into the rest of the flour-butter mixture, stirring to blend. Return this mixture to the top of the double boiler over boiling water. Cook, stirring constantly, until the mixture thickens.
4. To assemble the moussaka, line the bottom of an ovenproof baking dish with rounds of

eggplant; cover with a layer of the meat mixture; add another layer of eggplant rounds, followed by the rest of the meat mixture. Cover this with the white sauce; sprinkle it with the grated cheese. Place in a 350-degree oven and bake until the top has browned and the mixture has thoroughly cooked through, about 45 minutes.

YIELD: Serves 12
SODIUM CONTENT: 119 mg. of sodium per serving

VEALBURGERS

INGREDIENTS
- 1 1/2 lbs. ground veal
- 2 tbsp. fresh horseradish or low-sodium prepared horseradish
- 2 tbsp. finely chopped red onion
- 1 tbsp. finely chopped parsley
- dash of ground sage
- dash of salt-free garlic powder
- freshly ground black pepper to taste

DIRECTIONS:
1. Combine all the ingredients in a bowl, working the horseradish, onion, and spices into the meat with your fingers. Form into patties, place on a plate, cover with plastic wrap, and allow to stand for about 20 minutes so that the flavors combine. Cook over the charcoal grill, or broil or pan-fry as you would hamburgers.

YIELD: 6 burgers
SODIUM CONTENT: 78 mg. of sodium per burger

CHILI CON CARNE

- **Ingredients**
- 2 tbsp. olive oil
- 2 medium onions, chopped
- 1 medium green pepper, seeded and chopped
- 1 jalapeño or serrano pepper, seeded and minced
- 3/4 lb. lean ground beef
- 3/4 lb. ground pork
- 3 tbsp. salt-free chili powder
- 2 tbsp. ground cumin
- 1 tbsp. white wine vinegar
- 4 c. chopped fresh or salt-free canned tomatoes

- 1 bay leaf
- freshly ground black pepper to taste
- 15-oz. can salt-free red kidney beans or 2 c. cooked beans

DIRECTIONS:

1. Heat the olive oil in a large skillet or Dutch oven. Add the onion, green pepper, and hot pepper and cook for several minutes, until the onions and peppers begin to soften. Add the meat, breaking it apart and stirring until it is evenly browned and well combined with the other ingredients. Sprinkle the meat with chili powder, cumin, and balsamic vinegar, and stir to blend. Add the tomatoes, bay leaf, and black pepper, and stir to combine. Bring the mixture to a boil, reduce the heat, and simmer over low heat for 20 minutes. Add the kidney beans, including the water in which they are packed, and simmer for another half hour. Serve with rice or salt-free bread.

YIELD: Serves 8
SODIUM CONTENT: 61 mg. of sodium per serving

X. VEGETABLES

TARRAGON ROASTED VEGETABLES

INGREDIENTS

- 2 bell peppers, seeded and cut into 1-inch squares
- 2 yellow squash cut into
- 1/2-inch rounds
- 2 zucchini cut into 1/2-inch rounds
- 1 medium eggplant cut into 1/2-inch rounds, then cut into semicircles
- olive oil
- freshly ground black pepper to taste
- 2 tbsp. chopped fresh tarragon
- 1 tbsp. butter

DIRECTIONS:

1. Heat the vegetable grill pan on the charcoal grill or the skillet on top of the stove to medium-high heat. Spread all the pieces of vegetables on a plate in one layer. Drizzle olive oil over them and season them with black pepper and tarragon. When the grill pan or skillet is hot, add the vegetables and cook, tossing them around so they don't burn. Cook until the vegetables are tender, but not mushy. Serve either hot or at room temperature.

YIELD: Serves 6
SODIUM CONTENT: 5 mg. of sodium per serving

RATATOUILLE

- **Ingredients**
- 1/2 c. olive oil
- 2 medium green peppers, seeded and diced
- 1 c. chopped onion
- 2 cloves garlic, minced
- 2 medium zucchini, diced
- 1 medium eggplant, diced
- 4 medium tomatoes
- 1 tbsp. dried basil or 2 tbsp. chopped fresh basil leaves
- freshly ground black pepper to taste

DIRECTIONS:

1. Heat 1/4 cup of the oil in a large skillet or heavy saucepan. Add the peppers, onion, and garlic, and sauté for about 5 minutes, until the onion is translucent and the peppers are tender. Remove and set aside. Heat 2 more tablespoons of oil, and add the zucchini. Cook for about 10 minutes, stirring frequently, until it becomes tender. Set aside the zucchini in a bowl and add the remaining 2 tablespoons oil to the pan. Add the eggplant and cook for about 5 minutes, until tender. Remove the cooked eggplant and combine with the cooked zucchini.

2. Cut the tomatoes into wedges, then cut each wedge in half. Return the cooked vegetables to the pan; add the tomatoes, basil, and ground pepper and stir to combine. Simmer over medium heat, stirring occasionally, until the vegetables cook down together, about 10 minutes. Serve hot or cold.

YIELD : Serves 6
SODIUM CONTENT: 10 mg. of sodium per serving

EGGPLANT AND PEPPERS

INGREDIENTS
- 1 small eggplant
- 3 sweet red peppers
- olive oil
- freshly ground black pepper to taste
- 8 fresh basil leaves, chopped
- 2 cloves garlic, minced
- 1 c. salt-free chickpeas

DIRECTIONS:

1. Preheat the oven to 350 degrees. Place the whole eggplant and peppers on a baking sheet, drizzle them with oil, and sprinkle them with pepper. Roast them in the oven for 45 minutes to 1 hour, until the eggplant is completely tender.
2. Remove them from the oven and drain off any excess oil. Heat 1 tablespoon of oil to medium heat in a skillet or in a sauté pan on top of the stove, and add the garlic. Allow it to cook for a few minutes, being careful not to let it burn. Add the chickpeas, stir to combine, and cook for several minutes until they are warmed through. Cut the eggplant and the peppers into 1-inch pieces, put them in a bowl, add the chickpea mix and basil, and stir to combine. Serve warm.

YIELD : Serves 8
SODIUM CONTENT: 4 mg. of sodium per serving

FRESH MOZZARELLA AND TOMATO NAPOLEON

- **Ingredients**
- 12 tbsp. olive oil
- 12 tbsp. balsamic vinegar
- 4 small balls (about 2 pounds) fresh unsalted mozzarella, sliced thin
- 1 bunch fresh basil
- 4 vine-ripe tomatoes, cut into 1/4-inch slices
- freshly ground black pepper to taste

DIRECTIONS:

1. Place six plates on the table. Drizzle 1 tablespoon of oil on each plate, followed by 1 tablespoon of vinegar. Place a slice of the cheese on each plate, then a basil leaf and then a slice of tomato. Repeat this process until all the slices of cheese and tomato are used up. Top each napoleon with another tablespoon of oil, another tablespoon of vinegar, and pepper to taste, and serve.

YIELD : Serves 6
SODIUM CONTENT: 8 mg. of sodium per serving

VEGETARIAN TERRINE

INGREDIENTS

- olive oil
- 1 large eggplant, sliced
- freshly ground black pepper to taste
- several slices salt-free fresh mozzarella cheese, about 3/4 lb.

- 2 medium yellow squash, sliced
- 2 medium zucchini, sliced
- 1 onion, diced
- 2 tomatoes, diced
- 2 tbsp. fresh chopped parsley
- 2 tbsp. fresh chopped basil
- pinch of thyme
- 1/2 c. grated low-sodium Gouda cheese

DIRECTIONS:

1. Wipe the bottom and sides of a deep ovenproof baking dish with olive oil. Place all of the eggplant in the dish, and sprinkle with olive oil and black pepper. Add a few mozzarella cheese slices. Make a second layer using yellow squash, oil, pepper, and cheese, and a third layer with zucchini, oil, pepper, and cheese.
2. Preheat the oven to 350 degrees. Mix the onion and tomato with the parsley, basil, and thyme, and spread them evenly over the top. Sprinkle with grated Gouda cheese. Cover loosely with aluminum foil and bake for 30 minutes. Then remove the foil and bake for another 10 minutes, or until cooked through.

YIELD : Serves 8

SODIUM CONTENT: 48 mg. of sodium per serving if made with Gouda cheese, 73 mg. with salt-free mozzarella

REFRIED BLACK BEANS

- **Ingredients**
- olive oil
- 1 medium onion, chopped
- 1 clove garlic, minced
- 1 jalapeño pepper, minced
- 2 (15-oz.) cans salt-free black beans or 4 c. cooked black beans
- 1 tbsp. ground cumin
- 1 tbsp. cider vinegar
- several slices unsalted Gouda cheese (optional)
- fresh cilantro leaves

DIRECTIONS:

1. Heat 2 tablespoons of oil in a large skillet with a cover. Add the onion, garlic, and jalapeño pepper, and cook uncovered over medium heat for several minutes, until the onion begins to turn golden brown. Drain the beans and reserve 1 cup of the liquid from the cans or cooking

pot. Add the beans to the skillet, 1 cup at a time, mashing them with a fork and stirring them into the onion mixture. Continue to add and mash the beans until all are mashed and well mixed with the onions, garlic, and pepper.

2. Add the cumin and vinegar to the liquid from the beans and stir. Pour this mixture over the beans in the skillet, and stir to blend. Continue to cook over medium heat, stirring occasionally to prevent burning, until the liquid cooks down and the mixture begins to thicken. Turn off the heat and allow the refried beans to stand for 5 minutes; they will thicken more as they cool. Then spread the cheese on top of the beans, cover the skillet, and turn on the heat again to medium. Heat for just a few minutes, until the cheese melts. Sprinkle each serving with fresh cilantro leaves.

YIELD : Serves 4
SODIUM CONTENT: 65 mg. of sodium per serving

FRIED GREEN TOMATOES

- **Ingredients**
- 1/2 c. flour
- 1/2 c. cornmeal
- freshly ground black pepper to taste
- 4 green tomatoes, cut into slices 1/4-inch thick
- 2 tbsp. vegetable oil
- lemon juice or lemon wedges

DIRECTIONS:

1. Combine the flour, cornmeal, and a generous grinding of pepper on a plate. Dip each tomato slice into the mixture so that it is evenly coated. Heat the oil in a skillet over medium heat. Add the tomato slices so that each lies flat on the bottom of the pan, and allow to cook about 2 minutes on one side, then turn and cook for another minute, or until tender. Remove to a plate lined with a paper towel to drain before serving. Sprinkle with lemon juice or serve with lemon wedges.

YIELD : Serves 4
SODIUM CONTENT: 17 mg. of sodium per serving

SAUTÉED MUSHROOMS

INGREDIENTS

- 1 tbsp. olive oil
- 2 tbsp. finely chopped onion
- 2 c. sliced mushrooms
- 1 tbsp. lemon juice

- 2 tsp. finely chopped fresh thyme
- freshly ground black pepper to taste

DIRECTIONS:

1. Heat the oil in a sauté pan and add the onion; cook for several minutes, until the onion turns translucent. Add the mushrooms and cook, stirring occasionally, until they wilt and give up their liquid. Sprinkle with the lemon juice, thyme, and pepper and cook for a few more minutes, stirring to make sure the lemon juice and pepper are well distributed. Serve immediately.

YIELD: 4 cups
SODIUM CONTENT: 2 mg. of sodium per 1/2-cup serving

ASPARAGUS WITH LEMON BROTH

- **Ingredients**
- 12 to 16 asparagus spears
- vegetable oil
- 1 shallot, minced
- 1 clove garlic, minced
- 1 c. low-sodium chicken broth
- juice of 1 lemon

DIRECTIONS:

1. Wash the asparagus spears and break off the tough, woody ends. Heat a small amount of oil over medium heat in a sauté pan large enough to hold all the ingredients. Add the shallot and garlic and cook for about 5 minutes. Then add the chicken broth, lemon juice, and sugar; stir to blend. Drop in the asparagus. Bring to a boil; reduce the heat to low, and simmer uncovered until the asparagus is just tender, about 8 to 10 minutes, depending on the thickness of the stalks. Remove the asparagus to a platter and pour the juice over it before serving.

YIELD: Serves 4
SODIUM CONTENT: 13 mg. of sodium per serving

SPAGHETTI SQUASH WITH VEGETABLE MARINARA

INGREDIENTS

- 1 large spaghetti squash (about 4 pounds), pierced with a fork
- 1 tbsp. olive oil
- 1 medium onion, diced

- 2 cloves garlic, chopped
- 1 small zucchini, sliced
- 1 yellow squash, sliced
- 4 medium tomatoes, chopped
- 1/4 tsp. dried basil
- 1/4 tsp. dried thyme
- 1/2 lb. white button mushrooms, sliced
- freshly ground black pepper to taste
- 1/2 c. white wine
- fresh parsley or cilantro for garnish
- grated low-sodium Gouda cheese

DIRECTIONS:

1. Preheat the oven to 350 degrees, and bake the whole spaghetti squash for 1 to 1 1/2 hours. It is ready when it feels tender inside when poked with a fork.
2. To make the sauce, heat the oil in a large saucepan; add the onion and garlic and cook for several minutes until the onion turns translucent. Add zucchini and yellow squash and cook for 5 minutes longer. Then add tomato, herbs, mushrooms, black pepper, and wine. Stir and let simmer, partially covered, for an hour (you can do this while the squash cooks). If the sauce cooks down too much, add a little water.
3. When the squash has cooked, remove it from the oven and cut it in half lengthwise. Scoop out the seeds; remove the stringy flesh and arrange the flesh on a platter in a large circle or oval with a depression in the middle. Pour the sauce into the middle of the squash, garnish with fresh parsley or cilantro, and serve, sprinkling grated Gouda cheese on each serving.

YIELD : Serves 8
SODIUM CONTENT: 25 mg. of sodium per serving

VEGETARIAN VINDALOO

INGREDIENTS

- olive oil
- 2 c. chopped onions
- 2 tsp. whole cumin seeds
- 2 tsp. mustard seeds
- 6 whole cloves
- 1 tbsp. cayenne pepper
- 2 tsp. paprika
- 2 tsp. turmeric

- 1 1/2 tsp. cinnamon
- 2 cloves garlic, finely minced
- 2 c. diced potatoes (1/2-inch cubes)
- 2 medium carrots, sliced (1/4-inch slices)
- 2 tbsp. salt-free tomato paste dissolved in 2 c. water
- 2 c. cauliflower florets
- 2 c. broccoli florets
- 1 medium eggplant cut into 1-inch cubes
- 2 tbsp. lemon juice
- 2 c. finely chopped tomatoes
- 1 medium zucchini, sliced thin (1/4-inch slices)
- 2 c. canned salt-free chickpeas or fresh chickpeas soaked overnight and cooked until tender
- 1/4 c. raisins
- 2 tbsp. cider vinegar

DIRECTIONS:

1. Heat 2 tablespoons olive oil in a heavy saucepan or Dutch oven, and add the onion. Cook for about 10 minutes over low-medium heat, stirring occasionally, until the onion begins to caramelize (turn brown as the natural sugar heats up). Meanwhile, use an electric spice grinder or a mortar and pestle to grind up the cumin seeds, mustard seeds, and cloves. Add them to the cayenne pepper, paprika, turmeric, and cinnamon and stir to blend.

2. When the onion has cooked, stir in the garlic and cook for a minute; then add the spice mixture and stir to blend. Add a bit more oil if the mixture seems too dry. Add the potatoes and carrots and 1 cup of the water-tomato paste mixture. Turn up the heat to bring the liquid to a boil; then turn it down so it simmers. Cook at a low simmer for about 7 minutes, then add the cauliflower and broccoli and cook for another 7 minutes.

3. While these vegetables are cooking, heat another tablespoon of oil in a skillet over medium heat and cook the eggplant in it, stirring to prevent burning, until it begins to soften. Sprinkle the eggplant with lemon juice. Add the eggplant, tomato, zucchini, chickpeas, and raisins to the main mixture and stir to blend. Pour the remaining tomato paste and water mixture over the vegetables. Add the vinegar, and simmer, covered, for another 10 minutes, until all the vegetables are tender and the flavors are fully developed. Serve with rice and plain yogurt.

YIELD : Serves 12
SODIUM CONTENT: 29 mg. of sodium per serving

STUFFED ACORN SQUASH

INGREDIENTS
- 1 medium acorn squash

- 2 tbsp. unsalted butter
- 1/2 c. chopped onion
- 1 c. chopped mushrooms
- 3 tbsp. chopped parsley
- freshly ground black pepper to taste
- juice of 1/2 lemon
- 1/2 c. salt-free bread crumbs
- 1 c. grated low-sodium cheese (Gouda or Swiss)

DIRECTIONS:

1. Preheat the oven to 350 degrees. Cut the squash in half lengthwise and scoop out the seeds. Place the halves cut side down in a baking pan, add a 1/2-inch of water, and bake in the oven for about 30 minutes, or until the squash is soft when pierced with a fork. While the squash is cooking, melt the butter in a frying pan, add the onion, and cook for several minutes until it turns translucent. Add the mushrooms, parsley, and pepper, and continue cooking for a few minutes. Stir in the lemon juice. Transfer the onion-mushroom mixture to a bowl. When the squash has cooked, remove it from the oven and scoop out most of the flesh, reserving the shells. Stir the cooked squash into the mushroom mixture.
2. Combine the bread crumbs and grated cheese. Add about half of this mixture to the squash-onion-mushroom mixture, and stir to blend. Divide the resulting mixture in half and spoon into the shells of the squash. Spread the remaining cheese-bread crumb mixture on top of the stuffed shells. Put them on a baking sheet and return them to the oven to cook for about 15 minutes, until the cheese has melted and they are heated through.

YIELD : Serves 2
SODIUM CONTENT: 42 mg. of sodium per serving

ITALIAN ZUCCHINI

- **Ingredients**
- 3 medium zucchini, thinly sliced
- 1/2 c. finely diced green pepper
- 1/2 c. finely chopped onion
- 1 clove garlic, minced
- 4 medium tomatoes, diced
- 1 tsp. oregano
- freshly ground black pepper to taste
- 1/2 c. grated low-sodium Gouda cheese
- **DIRECTIONS:**

1. Preheat the oven to 350 degrees. Put the zucchini slices in a casserole dish and stir in all the other ingredients except the cheese so that they are well distributed. Sprinkle the cheese over the top. Put the casserole in the oven and cook for about 45 minutes.

YIELD: Serves 6
SODIUM CONTENT: 23 mg. of sodium per serving

POTATO PANCAKES

INGREDIENTS
- 6 medium potatoes (about 2 pounds)
- 2 eggs
- 2 tbsp. milk
- 1 medium onion, finely chopped or grated
- 1 leek, finely chopped
- 2 tbsp. finely chopped parsley
- 1/2 c. flour
- 1 tbsp. lemon juice
- freshly ground black pepper to taste
- 2 tbsp. vegetable oil

DIRECTIONS:

1. Peel and wash the potatoes. Grate them on the coarse grid of a box grater. This will produce strands of potato about an inch long. Use a large knife to chop the potato into pieces about 1/8-inch long. Put the chopped potatoes in a large strainer or colander suspended over a bowl and press down on the potatoes to expel their juice. You may want to do this two or three times, allowing the potatoes to stand for a few minutes between each pressing.
2. Allow the juice to sit in the bottom of the bowl for a few more minutes so the potato starch collects at the bottom. Pour off the liquid so the starch remains at the bottom of the bowl.
3. Add the eggs and milk to the potato starch, and stir to combine. Then stir in the chopped onion, leek, parsley, and chopped potatoes. Add the flour and stir to combine; stir in the lemon juice and black pepper.
4. Heat the vegetable oil in a large skillet or on a griddle. Use a slotted spoon to lift about 1/4 cup of the potato mixture out of the bowl and press out excess moisture. Drop the batter into the skillet, and press with a spatula to make a pancake. Cook over moderate heat until golden brown on the bottom, then turn to brown the other side.
5. As the pancakes cook, remove them to a plate lined with a paper towel to drain off excess oil, and put the plate in a warmed oven while you finish cooking enough pancakes for the meal. Serve as soon as possible after cooking.

YIELD: 8 medium pancakes

SODIUM CONTENT: 28 mg. of sodium per pancake

HOT PEPPER PANCAKES

INGREDIENTS

- 2 tbsp. olive oil
- 1/2 sweet red pepper, seeded and minced
- 1/2 jalapeño or serrano pepper, seeded and minced
- 1/2 c. white flour
- 1/2 c. cornmeal
- 2 tsp. low-sodium baking powder
- 1 egg
- 1 c. milk
- 1 tbsp. salt-free chili powder

DIRECTIONS:

1. Heat 1 tablespoon of the oil in a skillet and cook the red and hot pepper in it over moderate heat until the red pepper softens. Mix the flour, cornmeal, and baking powder together in a bowl. Beat the egg lightly with a whisk, and stir in the milk. Add the egg-milk mixture to the dry ingredients and stir until they are moistened. Then stir in the peppers and the chili powder. Heat the remaining tablespoon of oil on a griddle or large frying pan and drop spoonfuls of the batter on it; when bubbles form at the edges, turn and cook the other side until cooked through. Keep warm until ready to serve.

YIELD : 8 pancakes

SODIUM CONTENT: 24 mg. of sodium per pancake

SCALLION PANCAKES

INGREDIENTS

- 2 tbsp. butter
- 1 1/2 c. chopped scallions
- 1/4 c. dry vermouth
- freshly ground black pepper to taste
- 1/2 c. whole-wheat flour
- 1/2 c. white flour
- 2 tsp. low-sodium baking powder
- 1 egg
- 1 c. milk
- 1 tbsp. vegetable oil

DIRECTIONS:
1. Heat the butter in a sauté pan over medium heat. Add the scallions and cook until they begin to soften. Add the vermouth and pepper; stir to blend, and allow the mixture to cook down for a few minutes. Remove from the heat and set aside. Combine the flours and baking powder in a bowl. In another bowl, beat the egg lightly with a whisk; stir in the milk and add this mixture to the dry ingredients. Stir until the dry ingredients are fully moistened. Pour equal amounts of the scallion mixture and the flour mixture into another bowl and stir briefly to blend. Heat the vegetable oil on a griddle or frying pan. Drop spoonfuls of the pancake batter onto the griddle; when bubbles appear at the edges, turn and continue to cook until cooked through.

YIELD : 8 pancakes
SODIUM CONTENT: 18 mg. of sodium per pancake

MUSHROOM PANCAKES

- **Ingredients**
- 1 tbsp. unsalted butter
- 2 c. finely minced cremini, porcini, or button mushrooms
- 1/4 c. chopped fresh parsley
- 1 tbsp. dried thyme or
- 2 tbsp. fresh thyme
- 1 tbsp. lemon juice
- freshly ground black pepper to taste
- 1/2 c. whole-wheat flour
- 1/2 c. white flour
- 2 tsp. low-sodium baking powder
- 1 egg
- 1 c. milk
- 1 tbsp. vegetable oil

DIRECTIONS:
1. Heat the butter in a sauté pan over medium heat. Add the mushrooms, parsley, and thyme. Cook until the mushrooms begin to soften; add the lemon juice and pepper, and stir to blend. Remove from the heat and set aside. Combine the flours and baking powder in a bowl. Beat the egg lightly with a whisk; stir in the milk, and add this mixture to the dry ingredients. Stir until the dry ingredients are fully moistened. Pour equal amounts of the mushroom mixture and flour mixture into another bowl and stir to blend. Heat vegetable oil on a griddle or frying pan; drop spoonfuls of the pancake batter onto the griddle; when bubbles appear at the edges, turn and continue to cook until cooked through.

YIELD : 8 pancakes
SODIUM CONTENT: 26 mg. of sodium per pancake

FRITTATA

- **Ingredients**
- 2 medium potatoes
- 3 tbsp. olive oil
- 1 clove garlic, minced
- 1 small onion, chopped
- 1/2 c. diced green pepper
- 1/2 c. diced tomato
- 1 tsp. dried basil or 2 tsp. fresh basil leaves
- juice of 1/2 lemon
- freshly ground black pepper to taste
- 6 eggs
- 1 c. fresh sweet corn or salt-free frozen corn
- 1/2 c. grated salt-free Gouda cheese

DIRECTIONS:

1. Peel the potatoes and put them in a pot to boil while you chop and dice the other vegetables. Boil the potatoes until they are not quite cooked through (a fork pushed into them resists at the center). Cut them into 1/2-inch cubes. Heat 2 tablespoons of the oil in a heavy metal frying pan on top of the stove. Add the garlic, onion, and green pepper and cook for several minutes until the onion is translucent. Add the tomato, basil, lemon juice, and a grinding of pepper; cook for another 5 minutes, stirring to prevent the mixture from sticking. Transfer to a bowl and allow to cool. Put the potatoes in the pan (add a little more oil if necessary) and cook, stirring occasionally, until tender. Add them to the other vegetables and stir.

2. Preheat the broiler. Beat the eggs together in a bowl and stir in the cooked vegetables along with the corn. Reheat the remaining oil in the pan and pour the egg-vegetable mixture back into it. Cook for several minutes, until the egg has almost cooked through (cooking time will vary depending on the diameter of the pan and the depth of the egg mixture). Sprinkle the cheese on top of the frittata and place it under the broiler for a few minutes, until the rest of the egg has cooked and the cheese has melted. Serve immediately.

YIELD : Serves 8
SODIUM CONTENT: 71 mg. of sodium per serving

ASPARAGUS FRITTATA

- **Ingredients**

- 6 asparagus spears
- 1/2 lemon
- 1 tbsp. unsalted butter
- 1 shallot, minced
- 6 eggs
- 1/4 c. milk
- freshly ground black pepper to taste
- 1/4 tsp. tarragon
- 2 plum tomatoes, diced

DIRECTIONS:

1. Cut the tips off the asparagus spears, then cut the tender part of the stalks into 1/4-inch pieces (discard the woody ends). Blanch the asparagus by immersing it for 5 minutes in 6 cups of simmering water with the half lemon. Strain, remove the asparagus to a bowl of ice water to stop the cooking, and drain. Melt the butter in an ovenproof sauté pan. Turn to medium heat; add the shallot and sauté for 6 minutes, then remove from the heat. Place the eggs in a bowl, add the milk and beat lightly, then stir in the black pepper and tarragon. Add the asparagus and diced tomato, and stir to blend.

2. Return the sauté pan with the shallots to the stovetop over low heat, and add the egg mixture. Cook on low until the eggs start to firm up. Then turn on the broiler and place the sauté pan under the broiler until the top of the frittata cooks through from the top. You can serve the frittata from the pan if you wish, or you can remove it by placing a plate on top of the pan and flipping it over, then placing another plate on the bottom of the frittata and flipping it back.

YIELD : Serves 8
SODIUM CONTENT: 61 mg. of sodium per serving

HORSERADISH MASHED POTATOES

INGREDIENTS

- 6 large potatoes, peeled and sliced into quarters
- 4 tbsp. (1/2 stick) unsalted butter
- 1 1/2 c. whole milk
- freshly ground black pepper to taste
- 4 tbsp. finely grated fresh horseradish root

DIRECTIONS:

1. Add the potatoes to a large pot filled with water, bring to a boil, and cook until the potatoes are very tender, about 25 minutes. Drain the potatoes in a colander, then return them to the pot with the butter. Use a hand mixer or a potato masher to mash the potatoes, slowly adding

the milk. When all the milk has been added, season with pepper, add the horseradish, and stir well to combine.

YIELD : Serves 6

SODIUM CONTENT: 40 mg. of sodium per serving

BASIL MASHED POTATOES

INGREDIENTS

- 6 or 7 large potatoes
- 10 to 12 fresh basil leaves
- 3 tbsp. unsalted butter
- freshly ground black pepper to taste
- 1 to 1 1/2 c. milk

DIRECTIONS:

1. Peel and cut up the potatoes; cover them with water in a large pot. Bring the water to a boil; boil until the potatoes are very soft or fork tender, about 25 minutes. While the potatoes are boiling, add the basil leaves and the butter to a food processor and blend until there are no lumps of butter and the basil is finely chopped. Stir in a grinding of pepper. When the potatoes are cooked, drain and add to the basil and butter. Start to blend, and add the milk gradually. Blend until the lumps are gone and the mixture is smooth. Serve hot or transfer to a 200-degree oven until ready to serve.
2. If you don't have a food processor, chop the basil leaves as finely as you can with a knife, then put them and the butter in with the potatoes and add the milk as you mash them by hand.

YIELD : Serves 6

SODIUM CONTENT: 39 mg. of sodium per serving

WHIPPED POTATOES WITH ROSEMARY AND ROASTED GARLIC

- **Ingredients**
- 1 whole head of garlic
- 2 tbsp. olive oil
- 6 large russet potatoes
- 1/2 c. (1 stick) unsalted butter
- 2 tbsp. finely chopped fresh rosemary
- freshly ground black pepper to taste
- 1 c. milk

DIRECTIONS:

1. Preheat the oven to 375 degrees. Place the whole head of garlic in an ovenproof baking dish, drizzle the oil over it, and roast it for an hour. While it is roasting, peel and wash the potatoes, and cut them into equal sized pieces. In a large pot add enough water to cover the potatoes; bring the water to a boil and cook the potatoes until fork tender. When the garlic has cooked, remove it from the oven and use a sharp knife to slice off about 1/4 inch of the pointed top. Then hold the garlic head over a small bowl and squeeze it so the cooked garlic oozes out like toothpaste.

2. When the potatoes are cooked, place the butter, garlic, rosemary, and a generous grinding of black pepper in a bowl large enough for all the ingredients. Drain the potatoes well and add them to the bowl. Use a hand mixer to whip the potatoes, incorporating the milk and blending the other ingredients. Serve warm.

YIELD: Serves 6
SODIUM CONTENT: 34 mg. of sodium per serving

POTATOES ROSTI

- **Ingredients**
- 2 lbs. (6 medium) potatoes
- 4 tbsp. unsalted butter
- 2 tsp. onion powder
- freshly ground black pepper to taste
- grated low-sodium Gouda or Swiss cheese
- sprigs of parsley

DIRECTIONS:

1. Peel the potatoes and boil or steam them until partially cooked, about 10 minutes. Use the coarse grid of a box grater to grate the potatoes until you have 4 cups. Melt 2 tablespoons of butter; pour the butter over the potatoes and stir to combine, then stir in the onion powder and black pepper. Melt the other 2 tablespoons of butter in a skillet over moderate heat. Put the potatoes in the skillet and use a spatula to press them flat. Reduce the heat to low and continue to cook for about 20 minutes, until a golden brown crust forms on the bottom of the potatoes. If you think it may be cooking too hard on the bottom (and you're not watching your cholesterol) work a bit more butter in around the sides of the pancake as it cooks.

2. When a nice crust has formed, slide a spatula underneath the pancake to loosen it. Then remove the skillet from the heat and place a large plate upside down over the skillet. Quickly flip the skillet over, holding the plate in place, so the pancake falls out onto the plate, crust side up. Sprinkle with the cheese and a few sprigs of parsley. To serve, cut in wedges.

YIELD: Serves 4
SODIUM CONTENT: 17 mg. of sodium per serving

SWEET POTATO SUPREME

- **Ingredients**
- 4 or 5 large sweet potatoes
- 2 tbsp. butter
- 1 shallot, finely chopped
- 3 tbsp. molasses
- freshly ground black pepper to taste
- 1 c. milk

DIRECTIONS:

1. Put the potatoes in the oven and roast at 350 degrees until tender. This could take as much as 1 1/2 hours or more, depending on the size of the potatoes. (If you wish, you can roast the potatoes a day before.) Leave them unpeeled until ready for use. Heat a small slice of butter in a sauté pan over medium heat. Add the shallot and cook until wilted, taking care not to burn it. Allow the potatoes and shallot to cool while the milk and the rest of the butter warm to room temperature. When everything is ready, remove the potato skins and place the potato flesh in a bowl. Add the rest of the ingredients and mash them together with a hand potato masher. Just before serving, heat the mixture in a 350 degree oven.

YIELD : Serves 6
SODIUM CONTENT: 34 mg. of sodium per serving

SWEET POTATOES, CARROTS, AND SQUASH

INGREDIENTS

- 1 tbsp. butter
- 4 large carrots, sliced into 1-inch pieces and steamed
- 3 sweet potatoes, baked and peeled
- 1 acorn squash, baked and peeled
- 1/2 tsp. nutmeg

DIRECTIONS:

1. Melt the butter in a sauté pan; add the steamed carrots, cooking for a few minutes so that they absorb the butter. Put the carrots, sweet potatoes, and squash in a food processor or blender and process until smoothly puréed. Transfer to a saucepan and stir in the nutmeg. Cook over moderate heat until heated through. Serve warm.

YIELD : Serves 6
SODIUM CONTENT: 24 mg. of sodium per serving

CHESTNUT CREAM

INGREDIENTS
- 1 lb. chestnuts
- 1 medium bulb fennel
- 1 c. plain yogurt

DIRECTIONS:
1. Use a sharp knife to cut a cross in the flat side of each chestnut, then immerse in boiling water for 5 minutes. Turn off the heat, retrieve the chestnuts one by one, and peel off the outer and inner shells. Put the chestnut meats in a steamer basket in a saucepan with a little water. Bring the water to a boil and allow the chestnuts to steam for about 10 minutes, until tender. Clean and dice the fennel bulb and steam it, separately from the chestnuts, until tender, about 10 minutes. Then put the chestnuts, fennel, and yogurt in a blender or food processor and process to create a smooth cream. Serve warm.

YIELD: Serves 4
SODIUM CONTENT: 47 mg. of sodium per serving

ONION TART

FOR THE CRUST:
- 1/2 c. (1 stick) plus 2 tbsp. cold unsalted butter or margarine
- 11/4 c. all-purpose flour
- 1 tsp. sugar
- 3 tbsp. ice water

FOR THE FILLING:
- 1 tbsp. butter
- 2 large onions, cut in half and sliced thin
- 1 c. heavy cream
- 2 eggs
- freshly ground pepper to taste

DIRECTIONS:
1. To make the crust, slice the butter into small pieces and put them in a food processor fitted with a metal blade. Combine the flour and sugar, add them to the food processor, and process until the butter and flour begin to mix. Dribble in the ice water while the processor continues to run. When the dough comes together in a ball, remove to a bowl, wrap in waxed paper, and refrigerate. (To make the dough by hand, combine the flour and sugar and cut them into the butter with a pastry blender, two knives, or your fingertips. Add the water and continue to mix until the dough clings together.)

2. To make the filling, heat the butter in a pan; add the onion, and cook over medium heat for 15 minutes, making sure not to burn the onion. The onions should caramelize, turning brown and sweet. While the onions are cooking, put the cream and eggs in a bowl; beat them together, and add a generous grinding of pepper. When the onions are cooked, allow them to cool down.

3. Preheat the oven to 375 degrees. Roll out the dough to form a circle less than 1/4-inch thick. Press it gently into a 9-inch pie tin and trim off any dough that hangs over the edges. When the onions have cooled off, add them to the cream and egg mixture, and stir to combine. Pour this filling into the pie shell, put it on the middle rack of the oven, and bake for 35 to 45 minutes, until a toothpick stuck in the mixture comes out clean.

YIELD : Serves 8
SODIUM CONTENT: 32 mg. of sodium per serving

MUSHROOM AND ONION QUICHE

Ingredients

FOR THE CRUST:

- 1/2 c. (1 stick) plus 2 tbsp. cold unsalted butter or margarine
- 11/4 c. all-purpose flour
- 1 tsp. sugar
- 3 tbsp. ice water

FOR THE QUICHE:

- 1 tbsp. butter
- 1 onion, diced
- 2 c. sliced white button mushrooms
- 4 eggs
- 1 c. milk
- 1 c. heavy cream
- pinch of nutmeg
- freshly ground black pepper to taste

DIRECTIONS:

1. To make the crust, slice the butter into small pieces and put them in a food processor fitted with a metal blade. Combine the flour and sugar, add them to the food processor, and process until the butter and flour begin to mix. Dribble in the ice water while the processor continues to run. When the dough comes together in a ball, remove to a bowl, wrap in waxed paper, and refrigerate. (To make the dough by hand, combine the flour and sugar and cut them into the butter with a pastry blender, two knives, or your fingertips. Add the water and continue to mix until the dough clings together.)

2. To make the quiche, melt the butter in a frying pan over medium-high heat; add the onion and cook for 5 minutes. Add the mushrooms and cook for another 7 to 10 minutes until they release their liquid. While the mushrooms and onions are cooking, beat the eggs in a bowl and add the milk and heavy cream. Stir in the nutmeg and pepper.

3. Preheat the oven to 350 degrees. Roll out the dough to line a 9-inch pie tin. Bake the crust for 15 minutes. While the crust bakes, remove the mushroom mixture from the frying pan and let cool. Spread the cooled mushroom mixture in the baked crust. Then pour the egg mixture over the mushrooms and bake for about 40 minutes, until the top is golden brown. Test for doneness by sticking a knife in the middle of the custard mixture. When it comes out clean, the quiche is done.

YIELD: Serves 8
SODIUM CONTENT: 63 mg. of sodium per serving

BRUSCHETTA

INGREDIENTS
- 4 slices salt-free bread
- good quality olive oil
- 2 medium tomatoes, seeded and cut into 1/2-inch cubes
- 1 tbsp. balsamic vinegar
- 1 tsp. lemon juice
- freshly ground black pepper to taste
- 1 whole clove garlic, peeled
- 4 slices low-sodium Gouda or fresh salt-free mozzarella cheese (about 6 oz. altogether)
- 4 fresh basil leaves

DIRECTIONS:
1. Put the slices of bread on a baking sheet and place them under the broiler until lightly toasted. Turn them over and brush the untoasted side with olive oil, then return them to the broiler until that side is lightly toasted. Meanwhile, combine the tomatoes, balsamic vinegar, and black pepper in a bowl and stir to blend.

2. Rub the clove of garlic over the oiled, toasted slices of bread, then spoon equal portions of the tomato mixture onto each one. Top each one with a slice of cheese and return to the broiler just long enough to melt the cheese. Place a fresh basil leaf on top of each bruschetta before serving.

YIELD: Serves 4
SODIUM CONTENT: 24 mg. of sodium per serving if Gouda cheese is used, 69 mg. with fresh mozzarella

EGG NOODLES WITH PEAS AND GARLIC DRESSING

- **Ingredients**
- 1/2 c. low-sodium chicken broth
- 1 1/2 c. fresh or salt-free frozen peas
- 1 tbsp. unsalted butter
- 1 small shallot, finely chopped
- 4 cloves garlic, finely minced
- 1 pound egg noodles, cooked without salt and drained
- freshly ground black pepper to taste
- 2 tbsp. chopped parsley

DIRECTIONS:

1. Heat the chicken broth and peas in a saucepan; bring to a boil and cook until the liquid is almost gone. Add the butter, shallot, and garlic and cook for 5 minutes. Add the egg noodles. Stir to combine, and cook until heated through. Sprinkle with the pepper and chopped parsley; stir and serve.

YIELD: Serves 4
SODIUM CONTENT: 19 mg. of sodium per serving

ASPARAGUS AND SPINACH WITH PASTA

- **Ingredients**
- 2 tbsp. olive oil
- 2 cloves garlic, minced
- 1 medium sweet red pepper, seeded and diced
- 5 c. raw spinach leaves, stems removed, packed
- 12 stalks asparagus
- 2 tbsp. balsamic vinegar
- freshly ground black pepper to taste
- grated low-sodium Swiss or Gouda cheese
- 1 lb. linguini, ziti, or small shells cooked without salt and drained

DIRECTIONS:

1. Heat the oil in a large skillet, and add the garlic and sweet pepper. Cook over medium heat,

stirring occasionally, until the pepper softens. Add the spinach leaves and stir to combine. Cover and reduce the heat to very low as the spinach cooks down. Meanwhile, cut off the tips of the asparagus, then cut the rest of each stalk into 1-inch lengths, discarding the tough, woody ends. Put the pieces of asparagus in a steamer basket in a saucepan over an inch of water; bring to a boil, cover, and steam for about 5 minutes, until the asparagus turns bright green. It should be tender but still a bit crunchy. Combine the steamed asparagus with the spinach mixture; sprinkle with the balsamic vinegar and pepper, and toss to blend. Serve over linguini, ziti, or small shells sprinkled with grated cheese.

YIELD : Serves 4
SODIUM CONTENT: 67 mg. of sodium per serving

SHRIMP WITH PASTA AND PESTO

- **Ingredients**
- 2 tsp. olive oil
- 1 lb. shrimp, shelled and deveined
- 2 cloves garlic, finely chopped
- 1/2 c. white wine
- 1/4 c. plus 1 tbsp. salt-free pesto
- 1/2 c. low-sodium chicken broth
- 1 lb. pasta cooked without salt and drained

DIRECTIONS:

1. Heat the oil in a pot large enough to hold all the ingredients. Add the shrimp and garlic and cook for 2 minutes, then remove the shrimp from the pot. Add the wine and deglaze, using a wooden spoon to scrape bits of shrimp and garlic from the bottom of the pot. Then add the pesto and the chicken broth, and cook until it starts to simmer. Add the pasta and toss together. To serve, spoon pasta onto a plate, then arrange several shrimp on top of it.

YIELD : Serves 4
SODIUM CONTENT: 179 mg. of sodium per serving

CHICKEN AND PASTA SALAD WITH VEGETABLES

INGREDIENTS

- 1 lb. elbow macaroni, ziti, or other small pasta
- 1 c. olive oil
- 1 boneless chicken breast (2 half breasts)
- 2 tbsp. fresh thyme or 1 tbsp. dried thyme

- freshly ground black pepper to taste
- 3 medium carrots, peeled and cut into 2-inch strips
- 1 yellow sweet pepper, seeded and cubed
- 1 red sweet pepper, seeded and cubed
- 1 medium zucchini, cut into julienne strips
- 12 stalks asparagus, washed and cut into 2-inch pieces
- 1 jalapeño or serrano pepper, minced
- 1/4 c. balsamic vinegar
- 3 cloves garlic, minced
- juice of 1/2 lemon

DIRECTIONS:

1. Cook the pasta according to the **DIRECTIONS** on the package, omitting salt. Drain and toss with a little of the olive oil, and transfer to a large bowl to cool. Preheat the oven to 350 degrees. Brush the chicken with olive oil and sprinkle with 1 tablespoon of the fresh thyme (1 teaspoon dried) and black pepper. Place in an ovenproof pan or dish and roast in the oven until cooked through, about 1/2 hour. Remove and allow to cool.

2. Meanwhile, steam the carrots, peppers, zucchini, and asparagus one at a time until tender. Cut the chicken into thin 2-inch strips; add to the pasta and stir to combine. Then stir in the steamed vegetables, one at a time. Sprinkle the minced hot pepper over the mixture and stir once more.

3. Prepare the dressing by whisking together the remaining olive oil, vinegar, garlic, and the rest of the thyme. Pour this mixture over the pasta-chicken mixture and stir. Sprinkle with black pepper and lemon juice and stir once more. If you wish, add a bit more vinegar, lemon juice, or black pepper to taste before serving.

YIELD : Serves 6
SODIUM CONTENT: 44 mg. of sodium per serving

STUFFED SHELLS WITH SPINACH AND PARSLEY

INGREDIENTS
FOR THE SAUCE:

- 1 tbsp. olive oil
- 1/2 medium onion, chopped
- 1 clove garlic, minced
- 2 c. salt-free canned tomatoes or coarsely chopped fresh tomatoes
- 2 tbsp. red wine

- 1 tsp. balsamic vinegar
- 1 tsp. lemon juice
- 1 tsp. dried basil or 2 tsp. chopped fresh basil leaves
- 1/2 tsp. sugar
- freshly ground black pepper to taste

FOR THE SHELLS:
- olive oil
- 1/2 medium onion, chopped
- 1 clove garlic, minced
- 2 c. raw spinach
- 1 c. parsley leaves, tightly packed
- juice of 1/2 lemon
- 1 c. mascarpone cheese
- 1 c. plain yogurt
- 24 large pasta shells
- 3 to 4 tbsp. grated low-sodium Gouda cheese

DIRECTIONS:

1. To make the sauce, heat the olive oil in a heavy saucepan. Add the onion and garlic, and cook over medium heat until the onion begins to wilt. Add the rest of the sauce ingredients, bring to a simmer, and cook for at least an hour. If you prefer a smooth sauce, transfer the cooked mixture to a blender or food processor and process until smooth.

2. To make the filling, heat 1 tablespoon of olive oil in a sauté pan. Add the onion and garlic, and cook over medium heat until the onion begins to wilt. Then add the spinach and cook, stirring, until the spinach cooks down to about half its volume. Add the parsley and lemon juice, and cook for a few more minutes until the parsley softens. Transfer this mixture to a food processor or blender, and process briefly so that all the ingredients are chopped fine and well distributed. Combine the mascarpone and yogurt in a bowl, add the spinach-parsley mixture and stir until well blended.

3. Preheat the oven to 350 degrees. Cook the shells according to package **DIRECTIONS** (omitting salt) until they just begin to turn tender. Don't overcook, since they will cook more when filled. Lightly oil the bottom of a baking dish with olive oil. Drain the shells and fill each one with a spoonful of the spinach-parsley mixture. Place them seam side up in the baking dish. Pour the tomato sauce over and around the shells, then sprinkle the whole dish with grated cheese. Cover loosely with aluminum foil and bake until the cheese has melted and the shells are heated through, about 20 minutes.

YIELD: Serves 6

SODIUM CONTENT: 67 mg. of sodium per serving

CHICKEN AND SUN-DRIED TOMATOES WITH PASTA

INGREDIENTS

- 8 ounces elbow macaroni, ziti, or other small pasta
- 2 boneless chicken breasts (4 half breasts)
- 2 tbsp. olive oil
- 4 cloves garlic, minced
- 1/2 tsp. salt-free chili powder
- juice of 1/2 lemon
- freshly ground black pepper to taste
- 3 c. low-sodium chicken broth
- 1/2 c. chopped parsley
- 1/2 c. reconstituted dried tomatoes (20 tomato halves), cut into small pieces
- 8 green onions, chopped

DIRECTIONS:

1. Cook the pasta according to package **DIRECTIONS**, omitting salt. Rinse the chicken breasts, trim off any fat and skin, and cut the flesh into strips about 1/2 inch wide and 2 inches long. Heat the olive oil to medium in a large sauté pan or skillet, add the garlic, and cook for a few minutes until it softens. Add the chicken and cook for a few more minutes, until cooked through. Sprinkle with chili powder, lemon juice, and black pepper, and stir to blend. Remove the chicken from the pan and set aside.

2. Add the chicken broth, parsley, tomatoes, and green onions to the pan; bring to a boil and allow to cook down for several minutes, until the liquid is reduced by a third or more. Then return the chicken to the pan; stir. Cook for a few more minutes so that the flavors are well blended. Put the pasta in a large bowl, pour the sauce over it, and stir to combine before serving.

YIELD : Serves 6
SODIUM CONTENT: 81 mg. of sodium per serving

RISOTT O

INGREDIENTS

- 1 tbsp. unsalted butter
- 3 whole cloves garlic
- 1 shallot, finely chopped
- 6 medium mushrooms, sliced

- 1 1/2 c. arborio rice
- 5 to 6 c. salt-free chicken broth or water
- 1/4 c. grated salt-free Gouda cheese
- freshly ground black pepper to taste

DIRECTIONS:

1. Put the butter, garlic, shallot, and mushrooms into a deep pot and sauté over medium heat for 5 minutes or so. Add the rice and 2 cups of the broth or water and stir to combine. As the mixture cooks down add a cup at a time of the remaining broth or water until the rice is done. This will take about 30 minutes. After 20 minutes, add the cheese and stir until smooth. Add freshly ground pepper to taste and serve immediately.

YIELD : Serves 6
SODIUM CONTENT: 34 mg. of sodium per serving

BASIL RISOTTO

- **Ingredients**
- 2 tbsp. unsalted butter
- 1/2 shallot, finely diced
- 1 c. arborio rice
- 3 to 4 c. low-sodium chicken broth or water
- freshly ground black pepper to taste
- 10 basil leaves, finely chopped

DIRECTIONS:

1. Heat a pot to medium heat; add 1 tablespoon of the butter and the shallot. Cook for 5 minutes, then add the rice, stirring to coat the rice with the butter. Continue to cook for 6 minutes or so, making sure not to let the rice burn. Then add 1 cup of the chicken broth or water. Stir in the liquid, bring to a simmer, and cook until reduced by at least half. Add 1/2 cup of the liquid, bring to a simmer again, and allow to cook down; repeat this process until the rice is soft and the liquid is almost gone. The rice should have a creamy appearance and texture. This may occur before all of the liquid is used up—if the rice has a good texture after adding 2 1/2 or 3 cups of liquid, don't continue to add more. Finally, add the pepper, basil, and the rest of the butter, stir until the butter is incorporated. Serve immediately.

YIELD : Serves 4
SODIUM CONTENT: 33 mg. of sodium per serving

ROASTED TOMATO RISOTTO

- **Ingredients**
- 2 tomatoes, halved and seeded

- 1 clove garlic, sliced
- 2 tbsp. olive oil
- freshly ground black pepper to taste
- 2 tbsp. unsalted butter
- 1 shallot, minced
- 1 1/2 c. arborio rice
- 5 to 6 c. low-sodium chicken broth
- 6 basil leaves, chopped

DIRECTIONS:

1. Preheat oven to 400 degrees. Place the tomato halves cut side up on a baking sheet, and put two slices of garlic in each half. Drizzle oil over the tomatoes and sprinkle them with pepper. Roast them in the oven for 25 minutes. While the tomatoes are roasting, heat up a pot large enough for the risotto on top of the stove. Add 1 tablespoon of unsalted butter to the pot; add the shallot and cook for about 8 minutes, until thoroughly wilted. Add the rice and the other tablespoon of butter; stir to blend, and cook until the butter has melted. Add enough of the chicken broth just to cover the rice, and reduce the heat to low. When the broth has cooked down, add more, allow it to cook down, and repeat until the rice is soft.
2. When the tomatoes are roasted, remove them from the oven and allow them to cool to the point where you can easily handle them. Cut them up, add them to the rice with the basil, and stir to blend. Serve hot.

YIELD : Serves 6
SODIUM CONTENT: 36 mg. of sodium per serving

CARAMELIZED ONION RISOTTO

- **Ingredients**
- 2 tbsp. unsalted butter
- 1 leek, white part only, rinsed and finely chopped
- 1 small onion, finely chopped
- freshly ground black pepper to taste
- 1 1/2 c. arborio rice
- 5 to 6 c. low-sodium chicken broth

DIRECTIONS:

1. In a pot large enough for all the ingredients, melt 1 tablespoon of the butter over medium heat; add the leek and onion. Season with pepper, and cook over medium to low heat for about 15 minutes, stirring to prevent burning. The onion should turn golden brown. Add the rice and the second tablespoon of butter. Stir the rice to coat evenly with melted butter. Add 1 cup of broth and allow it to cook down slowly over low heat. When it is almost completely

absorbed, add another cup, repeating this process until rice is tender. If the rice seems to need more liquid, add a cup of water.

YIELD : Serves 6

SODIUM CONTENT: 35 mg. of sodium per serving

RISOTTO WITH ACORN SQUASH, SAGE, AND CHICKEN

- **Ingredients**
- 1 1/2 tbsp. unsalted butter
- 2 pinches allspice
- 1 acorn squash, cut in half, seeds removed
- 1 boneless chicken breast (2 half breasts)
- 1/2 shallot, finely minced
- 1 1/3 c. arborio rice
- 5 to 6 c. water or low-sodium chicken broth
- 8 fresh sage leaves, finely chopped
- freshly ground black pepper to taste

DIRECTIONS:

1. Preheat the oven to 375 degrees. Place 2 small slices of the butter on a baking sheet and sprinkle a pinch of allspice on each. Cover each piece of butter with a half of the squash, cut side down, and roast in the oven for 45 minutes to 1 hour, until very soft. While the squash is roasting, prepare the chicken. Trim the skin and fat off the breasts and cook them either by sautéing in a little oil over medium heat on top of the stove or by putting them on a baking sheet and baking them in the oven. Be sure they are cooked through.

2. In a large pot heat the rest of the butter; add the shallot and cook for several minutes, until it begins to soften. Add the rice and cook for another 4 minutes or so, stirring so the rice doesn't burn. Add just enough water or chicken broth to the pot to cover the rice. Allow to simmer uncovered, stirring every couple of minutes. When the liquid is absorbed, add another cup, repeating this process until the rice is tender.

3. When the rice is cooked, remove it from the heat and add sage, chicken, and black pepper. Scoop the flesh from the squash—it should be soft and creamy—and add it to the mixture; stir to incorporate. Serve in bowls, garnished with fresh sage.

YIELD : Serves 6

SODIUM CONTENT: 55 mg. of sodium per serving

LENTILS, RICE, AND ONIONS

- **Ingredients**
- 1 c. white rice
- 1 c. lentils
- 4 c. salt-free chicken broth
- 2 tbsp. olive oil
- 2 c. chopped onion
- 1/4 tsp. salt-free chili powder
- 1 tsp. lemon juice
- 1/2 tsp. ground cumin
- freshly ground black pepper to taste
- **DIRECTIONS**:

1. Put the rice and lentils in separate saucepans, and cover each with 2 cups of chicken broth. Bring both pans to a boil, reduce to a simmer, and cook until the rice and the lentils are just tender (about 15 minutes). Meanwhile, heat the oil in a large skillet or sauté pan, add the onions and cook, stirring occasionally, until they turn a deep brown and develop a full, sweet flavor.

2. Preheat the oven to 350 degrees. When the lentils are cooked, sprinkle them with the chili powder, lemon juice, and cumin, and stir to blend. When the rice is cooked, sprinkle it with a generous grinding of black pepper, and stir to blend. To assemble the final dish, stir the rice and lentils together in an ovenproof casserole. Press the rice and lentils down to create a flat surface, then spread a thick layer of onions on top of it. Place the dish on the middle rack of the oven and bake until the flavors develop, about 15 minutes. Serve warm.

YIELD : Serves 6
SODIUM CONTENT: 31 mg. of sodium per serving

ORZO WITH SUMMER VEGETABLES

- **Ingredients**
- 1 tbsp. unsalted butter
- 1 tbsp. corn oil
- 2 medium zucchini, diced
- 2 medium yellow
- squash, diced
- 1 red bell pepper, diced
- 1 small red onion, diced
- freshly ground black pepper to taste

1 lb. orzo cooked according to package **DIRECTIONS**, without salt, and drained

- 1/4 c. chopped parsley

DIRECTIONS:

1. Heat the butter and oil in a large skillet over medium heat. Add zucchini, squash, red pepper, and onion. Season with black pepper. Cook, stirring occasionally, for about 12 minutes. Remove the vegetable mixture from the heat and combine with the cooked orzo in a large bowl. Add the parsley and toss. Serve warm or cool.

YIELD: Serves 6
SODIUM CONTENT: 25 mg. of sodium per serving

BASIC TOMATO SAUCE

- **Ingredients**
- 2 tbsp. olive oil
- 1 medium onion, chopped
- 2 carrots, finely diced
- 1/2 tsp. dried thyme or 3 to 4 sprigs of fresh thyme
- 4 cloves garlic, chopped
- 1 c. red wine
- 10 fresh basil leaves, chopped
- 1 bunch parsley, roughly chopped
- 2 (15-oz.) cans salt-free whole tomatoes or 4 c. chopped fresh tomatoes
- freshly ground black pepper to taste

DIRECTIONS:

1. In a pot large enough for all the ingredients, heat the oil over medium-high heat. Add the onion and cook for several minutes, until it turns translucent. Add the carrots, thyme, and garlic, and cook for another 6 minutes. Add the wine, basil, parsley, and tomatoes, crushing the tomatoes with a wooden spoon or a potato masher. Stir well to combine. Season with pepper and simmer for 1 hour.

YIELD: Serves 4
SODIUM CONTENT: 24 mg. of sodium per serving

MEAT SAUCE FOR PASTA

- **Ingredients**
- 2 tbsp. olive oil
- 1 medium onion, chopped
- 4 cloves garlic, chopped
- 1 1/2 lbs. lean ground beef

- 2 tbsp. balsamic vinegar
- freshly ground black pepper to taste
- 2 (15-oz.) cans salt-free tomatoes or 4 c. chopped fresh tomatoes
- 1 bunch parsley, roughly chopped
- 8 fresh basil leaves, chopped, or 1 tbsp. dried basil
- 1 tbsp. fresh oregano leaves, or 1 tsp. dried oregano
- 1 c. red wine

DIRECTIONS:

1. Heat the oil in a large skillet or Dutch oven; add the onion and garlic and cook over medium heat for several minutes until the onion turns translucent. Add the meat and use a wooden spoon or potato masher to push it down so it cooks evenly. When the meat has browned, sprinkle it with the balsamic vinegar and black pepper, then stir to blend. Add the rest of the ingredients, stirring to blend. Allow the mixture to come just to a boil, then turn down to a low simmer and cook for an hour or more.

YIELD: Serves 8
SODIUM CONTENT: 67 mg. of sodium per serving

FRESH TOMATO SAUCE

INGREDIENTS

- 5 fresh, ripe tomatoes, seeded and diced
- 1/2 c. chopped fresh basil leaves
- 2 cloves garlic, minced
- 3 tbsp. olive oil
- 2 tsp. balsamic vinegar
- juice of 1/2 lemon
- 1/2 tsp. salt-free chili powder
- freshly ground black pepper to taste

DIRECTIONS:

1. Combine the diced tomatoes, basil, and garlic in a bowl and stir to distribute evenly; add the olive oil, vinegar, and lemon juice and stir to blend. Sprinkle with the chili powder and a generous grinding of black pepper. Stir again to blend, and allow to stand for at least 1/2 hour before serving.

YIELD: Serves 6
SODIUM CONTENT: 14 mg. of sodium per serving

GRILLED PEPPER AND TOMATO

SAUCE

- **Ingredients**
- 4 sweet red peppers
- 2 large ripe tomatoes, cut in half
- olive oil
- 1/2 red onion, finely chopped
- 1/4 c. chopped fresh parsley
- 2 tbsp. chopped fresh tarragon
- 8 basil leaves, chopped
- freshly ground black pepper to taste

DIRECTIONS:

1. Rub the peppers and tomatoes with olive oil and place over the charcoal grill or a medium open flame on top of the gas range. Let the skin of the peppers get black, then remove the peppers from the fire. Allow the tomatoes to grill only until they get a little mushy. When the peppers are cool enough to handle, remove the skin under cool water. Cut them into large chunks, and remove the membranes and seeds from the inside. Place the tomatoes and the peppers in a blender and blend to a smooth purée. Heat a tablespoon of oil in a saucepan over low to medium heat and sauté the onion in it for 10 minutes. Add the purée, along with the rest of the ingredients, and cook for about 45 minutes over low heat.

YIELD: Serves 4
SODIUM CONTENT: 15 mg. of sodium per serving

PASTA SAUCE WITH SUN-DRIED TOMATOES

- **Ingredients :**
- 16 salt-free sun-dried tomato halves
- 3 tbsp. olive oil
- 2 cloves garlic, minced
- 2 (15-oz.) cans salt-free tomatoes or 4 c. chopped fresh tomatoes
- 8 basil leaves, chopped
- juice of 1/2 lemon
- freshly ground black pepper to taste

DIRECTIONS:

1. Put the sun-dried tomatoes in a bowl, cover with boiling water, and set aside to soften for about 15 minutes. Heat the olive oil in a large sauté pan or pot. Add the garlic, and cook for 5

minutes over medium heat. Add the fresh tomatoes, basil, lemon juice, and pepper, and stir to blend. Bring the mixture to a simmer. When the sun-dried tomatoes have softened, remove them from the water, drain, and use a scissors or sharp knife to cut them into small pieces. Add the sun-dried tomatoes to the tomato mixture and allow to cook for another 20 minutes or so, until the liquids reduce and the flavors develop.

YIELD : Serves 6
SODIUM CONTENT: 21 mg. of sodium per serving

FESTIVE TOMATO SAUCE

- **Ingredients**
- 1 tbsp. olive oil
- 2 cloves garlic, minced
- 1 medium onion, chopped
- 2 (15-oz.) cans salt-free tomatoes or 4 c. chopped fresh tomatoes
- 1/4 c. red wine
- 2 tsp. balsamic vinegar
- 2 tsp. lemon juice
- 1 tsp. dried basil or 2 tsp. chopped fresh basil leaves
- 1 tsp. dried oregano or 2 tsp. fresh oregano leaves
- 2 tbsp. dried parsley or 1/4 c. chopped fresh parsley
- 1 large sprig fresh tarragon
- 1 tsp. sugar
- freshly ground black pepper to taste
- 3/4 c. fresh zucchini cut in 1-inch julienne strips
- 3/4 c. sliced fresh mushrooms
- **DIRECTIONS**:

1. Heat the olive oil in a heavy saucepan. Add the garlic and onion, and cook for several minutes, until the onion becomes translucent. Add the rest of the ingredients except for zucchini and mushrooms; stir to blend thoroughly and simmer, partially covered, for at least an hour. Then add zucchini and mushrooms and cook for no more than 15 minutes, so that zucchini strips remain al dente and retain their color.

YIELD : Serves 6
SODIUM CONTENT: 14 mg. of sodium per serving

PIZZA DOUGH

INGREDIENTS

- 2 packages or 4 1/2 tsp. dry yeast
- 2 c. lukewarm water
- 2 tbsp. olive oil
- 1 tbsp. honey
- 4-plus c. all-purpose flour

DIRECTIONS:

1. Dissolve the yeast in 1/2 cup of the water and allow to stand for a few minutes until it begins to foam. Add the oil, honey, and the rest of the water and stir to blend.

    Add 1 cup of flour, and stir. Add the rest of the flour, 1/2 cup at a time, stirring until the dough becomes too stiff to stir with a spoon. Remove it to a floured board and knead for about 5 minutes, until it feels soft and elastic and the texture is uniform.

2. (If you have a mixer with a dough hook, you can use it to knead the dough. After stirring in the first cup of flour by hand, put the mixture in the mixer's bowl, add 2 more cups of flour and run the mixer on slow speed. Add more flour 1/4 cup at a time until the dough holds together in a ball and no longer sticks to the sides of the bowl. After removing the dough from the bowl, knead by hand a few times to make sure the texture is uniform.)

3. Wipe the inside of a clean bowl with olive oil; place the dough in it to rise and cover loosely with plastic wrap. For a faster rise, put the bowl in a sink partly filled with hot water. The dough is ready to use for pizza crusts when it has doubled in bulk. There should be enough for four medium-sized pies.

YIELD: 24 slices
SODIUM CONTENT: less than 1 mg. of sodium per slice

BASIC PIZZA

INGREDIENTS

- salt-free pizza dough for one pie, risen once (1/4 of pizza dough recipe)
- cornmeal
- 1 c. salt-free tomato sauce
- 1/2 lb. salt-free fresh mozzarella cheese, sliced thin
- 1 tbsp. dried basil or 2 tbsp. chopped fresh basil leaves
- 1 tbsp. dried oregano or 2 tbsp. fresh oregano leaves
- 1 tbsp. high-quality olive oil
- 1/4 c. grated low-sodium Gouda cheese

DIRECTIONS:

1. Place a baking tile (if you have one) on the bottom rack of the oven and preheat it to 500 degrees.
2. Using first the heel of your palm, then your fingertips, flatten the ball of risen dough on a

floured board so that it forms a large circle no more than 1/4-inch thick. Forget the twirling and tossing of pizza parlor bakers; the best crusts are shaped by using the fingertips to push the edges of the dough out from the center of the circle.

3. Spread enough cornmeal across the surface of a baker's peel so the dough will slide off it easily. Transfer the flattened dough to the peel. (If you don't have a peel, transfer the dough to a large baking sheet lined with baker's parchment or spread with a thin layer of cornmeal.) Spread the tomato sauce evenly on the crust, followed by slices of the mozzarella cheese. Sprinkle with basil, oregano, and olive oil, then with the grated Gouda cheese. Be careful not to load the crust up with too much sauce and cheese, or it won't slide off the peel easily.

4. Open the oven door and carefully shift the pie to the baking tile, shoving the peel forward in short strokes so that the pie slides forward onto the tile. (If using a baking sheet, rest it on the tile. If you aren't using a tile, put the baking sheet on the bottom rack of the oven.) Close the door and cook the pie until the cheese bubbles on the surface and the edges of the crust turn dark brown, about 15 to 20 minutes. Slide the peel under the cooked pie and remove it from the oven. Cut into pieces with a sharp knife or a pizza wheel.

YIELD: 6 slices
SODIUM CONTENT: 62 mg. of sodium per slice

SPRING AND SUMMER PIZZA

- **Ingredients**
- 4 stalks fresh asparagus
- 1 large ripe tomato
- 1 medium summer squash
- 1 medium zucchini
- 1 medium onion
- 1 medium green pepper
- salt-free pizza dough for one pie, risen once (1/4 of pizza dough recipe)
- cornmeal
- 1 tbsp. olive oil
- 1 tbsp. dry basil or 2 tbsp. fresh leaves
- 1 tbsp. dry oregano or 2 tbsp. fresh leaves
- freshly ground black pepper to taste
- 1/4 lb. Swiss Lorraine cheese, sliced thin

DIRECTIONS:

1. Place a baking tile (if you have one) on the bottom rack of the oven and preheat it to 500 degrees. Cut the tough ends off the asparagus stalks and slice them lengthwise. Use a sharp knife to prepare paper-thin (if possible) slices of tomato, squash, zucchini, onion, and green

pepper.

2. Using first the heel of your palm, then your fingertips, flatten the ball of risen dough on a floured board so that it forms a large circle 1/4-inch thick. Spread enough cornmeal across the surface of a baker's peel so that the dough will slide off it easily. Transfer the flattened dough to the peel. (If you don't have a peel, transfer the dough to a large baking sheet lined with baker's parchment or spread with a thin layer of cornmeal.

3. Brush a thin layer of olive oil on the crust and arrange vegetable slices, in equal portions, on top of it. Do not use so many vegetable slices that they make the crust too heavy to slide easily off the peel. Sprinkle with basil, oregano, and ground pepper. Place slices of the cheese on the vegetables.

4. Open the oven door and carefully shift the pie to the tile, shoving the peel forward in short strokes so the pie slides forward onto the tile. (If using a baking sheet, rest it on the tile. If you aren't using a tile, put the baking sheet on the bottom rack of the oven.) Close the door and cook the pie until the cheese melts and the edges of the crust turn brown, about 15 to 20 minutes. Slide the peel under the cooked pie and remove it from the oven. Cut into pieces with a sharp knife or a pizza wheel.

YIELD : 6 slices
 SODIUM CONTENT: 28 mg. of sodium per slice

FRESH PIZZA

- **Ingredients**
- 2 medium ripe tomatoes, chopped
- 10 fresh basil leaves, chopped, or 2 tbsp. dried basil
- 1 tbsp. balsamic vinegar
- 1 clove garlic, finely minced
- freshly ground black pepper to taste
- olive oil
- salt-free pizza dough for one pie, risen once (1/4 of pizza dough recipe)
- cornmeal

DIRECTIONS:

1. Place a baking tile (if you have one) on the bottom rack of the oven and preheat it to 500 degrees. In a bowl, combine the tomatoes, basil, vinegar, garlic, a sprinkling of pepper, and 1 tablespoon of olive oil; stir to combine and set aside. Place the dough on a floured board and use your fingertips and the heels of your palms to flatten it into a large circle no more than 1/4-inch thick.

2. Transfer the flattened dough to a baking sheet lined with baker's parchment or spread with a thin layer of cornmeal. Brush a little olive oil on the crust, and place the baking sheet on the tile in the oven (or on the bottom rack if you don't have a tile). Bake for about 15 minutes,

until the crust turns golden brown and crisp.
3. To serve, cut the crust into sections with a sharp knife or pizza wheel and spoon a generous helping of topping onto each one. If the topping mixture seems too liquid, use a slotted spoon.

YIELD: 6 slices
SODIUM CONTENT: 5 mg. of sodium per slice

BERRY PIE

- **Ingredients**
- 3 1/2 c. fresh blueberries or raspberries
- 1/4 c. minute tapioca
- 1/2 c. sugar
- 1/2 c. water
- 2 tsp. lemon juice (if using blueberries)
- 9-inch precooked salt-free crumb or pastry crust

DIRECTIONS:
1. Put 2 cups of fresh berries along with all the remaining ingredients for the filling in a saucepan, stir to blend, and bring to a boil on top of the stove over medium heat. When the mixture reaches a full boil, remove it from the heat. Add the remaining 1 1/2 cups of fresh berries, and stir gently to distribute. The fresh berries will cook a bit and the mixture will thicken up as it cools. Allow to cool before pouring into the crust. If you want a top crust for a pie with a pastry bottom crust, bake strips or circles of pastry and float them on the filling. Sprinkle loose crumbs on a pie with a crumb crust.

YIELD: Serves 6
SODIUM CONTENT: 3 mg. of sodium per serving

AMARETTO CREAM PIE

INGREDIENTS
FOR THE CRUST:
- 1 1/2 c. amaretto cookie crumbs (about 17 cookies)
- 6 tbsp. unsalted butter or margarine, melted

FOR THE FILLING:
- 1/2 c. sugar
- 1/2 c. flour
- 2 c. milk
- 3 egg yolks, lightly beaten

- 1 tbsp. butter
- 1 tsp. vanilla

FOR THE MERINGUE:
- 2 egg whites
- 1/4 tsp. cream of tartar
- 2 tbsp. sugar
- 1/2 tsp. vanilla

DIRECTIONS:
1. Preheat oven to 350 degrees. To make crumbs for the crust, grind up cookies in a blender or food processor or crush them with a rolling pin between two sheets of waxed paper. Put the crumbs in a bowl and stir in the melted butter until thoroughly blended. Press the crumbs into a 9-inch pie tin, pushing them against the bottom and sides of the tin with your fingertips to form a crust of uniform thickness. Put the tin in the oven and bake for 10 minutes. Allow to cool before filling
2. To make the filling, put the sugar, flour, and milk in the top of a double boiler. Boil water in the bottom half and cook the sugar mixture over it until it begins to thicken. Remove it from the heat and pour half of it into a bowl containing the beaten egg yolks, stirring to blend. Then pour the egg mixture back into the rest of the sugar mixture and return it to cook over the boiling water, stirring until it thickens. Remove from the heat and add the butter and vanilla, continuing to stir until they are well blended. Allow the mixture to cool for a few minutes before pouring it into the amaretto crust.
3. When separating egg whites for the meringue, be extremely careful not to let any egg yolk contaminate the whites. If it does, the whites won't beat up into a thick meringue. To make meringue, beat the egg whites until they begin to foam; then add the cream of tartar and beat until they form stiff peaks that droop a bit as you pull the beater out of the bowl. Then stir in the sugar until thoroughly blended, followed by the vanilla.
4. Spread the meringue evenly on top of the cream filling, and put the pie in the oven to bake for about 10 minutes, until the peaks of the meringue are lightly browned.

YIELD: Serves 8
SODIUM CONTENT: 53 mg. of sodium per serving

LEMON CUPS

INGREDIENTS
- 1 c. sugar
- 1/4 c. all-purpose flour
- 2 tbsp. unsalted butter, melted
- 1/4 c. plus 1 tbsp. lemon juice

- rind of 1 lemon, finely grated
- 1 1/2 c. milk
- 3 egg yolks, beaten well
- 3 egg whites, beaten stiff

DIRECTIONS:

1. Preheat the oven to 350 degrees
2. Blend the sugar and flour and stir them together with the melted butter. Add the lemon juice and lemon rind and stir to blend. In a separate bowl, stir the milk into the beaten egg yolks. Then add the sugar-lemon-flour mixture to the eggs and milk and stir well. Fold in the beaten egg whites gently and evenly. Pour the mixture into 6 lightly greased ovenproof cups and place them in a shallow pan of hot water. Bake them for 45 minutes until the tops are golden brown.

YIELD : Serves 6
SODIUM CONTENT: 60 mg. of sodium per serving

BOURBON BREAD PUDDING

- **Ingredients**
- 4 c. salt-free white or whole-wheat bread cubes, crusts removed
- 2 3/4 c. warm milk
- 3 egg yolks
- 1/2 c. sugar
- splash of vanilla
- 1/4 c. bourbon

DIRECTIONS:

1. Preheat the oven to 350 degrees. Place the bread in a bowl and cover with warm milk. (Be sure the milk is warm and not hot, so you don't scramble the egg yolks you will be adding.) While the bread is soaking, mix the egg yolks with the sugar, and stir with a whisk until well combined. Add the vanilla and the bourbon, and whisk again. Add the yolk mixture to the bread, and stir to combine. Place the pudding in an ovenproof dish; place it in a larger pan, and add hot water to half the depth of the pudding dish. Put the whole thing in the oven and cook for 45 minutes.

YIELD : Serves 6
SODIUM CONTENT: 58 mg. of sodium per serving

RICE PUDDING

INGREDIENTS
- 1/2 c. long-grain rice

- 3 c. milk
- 1/2 c. sugar
- 1 tbsp. honey
- 1 tsp. cinnamon
- 2 large egg yolks
- 1/4 tsp. vanilla

DIRECTIONS:
1. Put the rice and milk in a saucepan and bring to a boil. Reduce the heat and simmer for 1 hour.
2. Combine the rest of the ingredients in a bowl and stir to blend. When the rice has cooked, add this mixture to it in small amounts, stirring constantly to avoid scrambling the egg yolks, and cook 5 minutes more until the pudding thickens. Pour the pudding into serving bowls, cover with plastic wrap, and refrigerate for 2 hours before serving.

YIELD: Serves 6
SODIUM CONTENT: about 64 mg. of sodium per serving

AMARETTO APPLE CRISP

INGREDIENTS
- 1 1/2 c. amaretto cookie crumbs (about 20 cookies)
- 6 c. peeled, cored, and thinly sliced apples
- 1 tsp. cinnamon
- 8 tbsp. (1 stick) butter
- 1/2 c. brown sugar
- 1/2 c. all-purpose flour
- 1/2 tsp. almond extract

DIRECTIONS:
1. Preheat the oven to 350 degrees. To prepare amaretto crumbs, grind up cookies in a blender or food processor or crush them with a rolling pin between two sheets of waxed paper. Put the apples in a bowl; add cinnamon, and stir until it is evenly distributed. Transfer the apples to a baking dish.
2. Cut the butter into small pieces and put them in a food processor. Add the sugar, flour, crushed cookies, and almond extract. Process for a few minutes until the mixture is thoroughly blended. (Or cut the butter into the rest of the ingredients in a bowl, using a pastry cutter, two knives, or your fingertips.) Spread the mixture over the apples and press it down into them to create a uniform crust. Bake on the middle rack of the oven until the crust has browned and the apples are cooked through, about 45 minutes. Allow to cool a bit before serving.

YIELD: Serves 8
SODIUM CONTENT: 12 mg. of sodium per serving

BLUEBERRY COBBLER

INGREDIENTS

FOR THE CRUST:
- 1 3/4 c. all-purpose flour
- 1 tbsp. sugar
- 1 tbsp. low-sodium baking powder
- 5 tbsp. chilled butter, cut into 1-inch pieces
- 3/4 c. heavy cream

FOR THE FILLING:
- 3 c. fresh or frozen blueberries
- 2/3 c. sugar
- 1 tbsp. flour

DIRECTIONS:

1. Preheat the oven to 425 degrees. To make the crust, sift the flour, sugar, and baking powder together in a bowl, and add the chilled butter. Combine the butter with the dry ingredients by squeezing the mixture gently through your fingers. When it consists of marble-sized balls, add the heavy cream, and continue to mix with your fingers only until the cream is absorbed. The dough should be crumbly, not smooth. Wrap in plastic wrap and refrigerate while you make the filling.

2. Heat the blueberries with the sugar and flour in a saucepan. Stir as the sugar melts; bring the mixture to a boil, then turn it off. Lightly grease a 9" × 9" ovenproof baking dish with butter. Add the berries and spread them out so that they cover the bottom of the dish. On a floured surface, roll out the dough just until it is large enough to cover the filling; the dough should be thick. Place the dough on top of the filling. Put the cobbler in the oven and bake for about 30 minutes, until the dough begins to brown. Allow to cool slightly before serving with vanilla ice cream.

YIELD: Serves 12
SODIUM CONTENT: 9 mg. of sodium per serving

APPLE WALNUT CAKE

INGREDIENTS
- 2 c. all-purpose flour
- 4 tsp. low-sodium baking powder
- 3/4 tsp. cinnamon

- 3/4 tsp. ground cloves
- 3/4 tsp. ground ginger
- 1/4 tsp. nutmeg
- 1 c. brown sugar, packed
- 1 c. plain yogurt
- 3/4 c. vegetable oil
- 1 egg
- 1 tsp. vanilla
- 2 tbsp. calvados
- 1 1/2 c. peeled, seeded, and chopped apples
- 3/4 c. chopped walnuts

DIRECTIONS:

1. Preheat the oven to 350 degrees. Lightly grease an 8" × 8" baking pan. In a large mixing bowl, combine the flour, baking powder, spices, and brown sugar, and stir to blend, making sure to break up any lumps in the sugar. In a separate bowl, stir together the yogurt and oil; add the egg, vanilla, and calvados. When this mixture is thoroughly blended, add the apples and walnuts, and stir to combine. Add the liquid mixture to the flour mixture and stir only until all the dry ingredients are moistened. Pour the batter into the baking pan, spreading it evenly with a rubber scraper. Bake on the middle rack of the oven for about an hour, or until a toothpick inserted into the center of the cake comes out clean.

YIELD: Serves 12
SODIUM CONTENT: 22 mg. of sodium per serving

ANGEL FOOD CAKE

INGREDIENTS

- 12 egg whites
- 1 tbsp. water
- 1 tsp. cream of tartar
- 1/2 tsp. vanilla
- 1/2 tsp. almond extract
- 1 1/2 c. sugar
- 1 c. cake flour

DIRECTIONS:

1. Preheat the oven to 350 degrees. Combine the egg whites, water, cream of tartar, vanilla, and almond extract in a large bowl; beat with an eggbeater or hand-held electric mixer until more than quadrupled in volume. Do not beat beyond the point where the whites form a soft foam.

Then continue to beat while adding 3/4 cup sugar in small amounts until the whites form soft peaks.

2. Sift together the cake flour and the remaining 3/4 cup sugar. Then sprinkle small amounts of this mixture over the egg whites, using a rubber scraper to fold the flour in each time. Fold gently and carefully; take care not to overmix.

3. Pour this mixture into an ungreased 10-inch tube pan, and spread gently so that it fills the pan evenly. Bake on the middle rack of the oven until a thin knife or bamboo skewer inserted into the middle of the cake comes out clean (about 35 minutes). Arrange three water glasses or jars in a triangle so they will support the rim of the pan when inverted. Set the pan upside down on the glasses and allow the cake to cool completely.

4. To remove the cake, run a thin knife around the circumference of the pan and of the tube without cutting into the cake. Then tap the pan on a hard surface and the cake should come out. If you have the kind of pan with a removable bottom, remove it with the cake and run the knife underneath the cake to separate it from the bottom of the pan.

YIELD : 12 slices

SODIUM CONTENT: 51 mg. of sodium per slice

PINEAPPLE UPSIDE-DOWN CAKE

INGREDIENTS

FOR THE GLAZE:

- 8 tbsp. (1 stick) unsalted butter or margarine
- 1/2 c. packed dark brown sugar
- 6 large slices (1/2-inch thick) of ripe fresh peeled pineapple with the fibrous core removed (or 8 to 10 canned pineapple rings)
- 24 pecan halves
- 2 tbsp. maple syrup

FOR THE CAKE BATTER:

- 1 c. sugar
- 3/4 c. unsalted butter or margarine
- 3 eggs
- 1 tsp. vanilla
- 1 more slice of fresh pineapple (or 2 canned rings)
- 3 c. all-purpose flour
- 1 tbsp. low-sodium baking powder
- 1 tsp. ground ginger

DIRECTIONS:

1. Preheat the oven to 350 degrees.

2. To prepare the glaze: Melt the butter or margarine and pour it into a 9" × 13" ovenproof baking dish. Add the brown sugar; stir to blend, and spread the mixture evenly across the bottom of the dish. Distribute the pineapple rings in two lines, pressing them into the sugar mixture. Press two pecan halves, curved side down, into the center of each ring, and distribute the others in the spaces between rings. Drizzle with the maple syrup.

3. To prepare the batter: Cream the sugar together with butter or margarine, and stir in the eggs and vanilla. Use a blender or food processor to grind up the single slice of fresh pineapple (or two slices of canned); add this purée to the butter-sugar-egg mixture and stir. Sift together the flour, baking powder, and ginger and add them to the liquid mixture, stirring to blend.

4. To assemble the cake: Pour the batter over the glaze in the baking dish, and use a rubber scraper to spread it to an even depth. Cook on the middle rack of the oven for 30 to 40 minutes until the cake has turned golden brown and a toothpick inserted into it comes out clean of batter (don't stick it all the way down to the glaze). Remove the cake from the oven and allow to cool for several minutes right side up. Run a knife around the edge to separate the cake from the sides of the dish. Place a tray or baking sheet large enough to cover the baking dish on top of it, then, using heavy potholders to protect your hands, quickly invert the baking dish and tap the bottom of it so that the cake drops onto the tray. If any glaze clings to the bottom of the baking dish, use a rubber scraper to remove it, and add it to the top of the upside-down cake. Serve warm.

YIELD: Serves 10
SODIUM CONTENT: 25 mg. of sodium per serving

GINGERBREAD

INGREDIENTS
- 1/4 c. unsalted butter, softened
- 1/4 c. vegetable shortening
- 1/4 c. dark brown sugar
- 1/4 c. white sugar
- 1 egg
- 1/4 c. molasses
- 2 c. flour
- 1 tbsp. low-sodium baking powder
- 2 tsp. ground ginger
- 2 tsp. cinnamon
- 1/2 tsp. ground cloves
- 3 tbsp. chopped crystallized ginger
- 1/2 c. boiling water

DIRECTIONS:
1. Preheat the oven to 350 degrees. Beat together the butter and shortening until thoroughly blended, then mix in the sugars, egg, and molasses. Sift together the flour, baking powder, ground ginger, cinnamon, and ground cloves. Add the dry ingredients to the liquid ingredients, stirring until just blended, then stir in the crystallized ginger. Add the boiling water and stir to blend. Lightly grease a 9-inch square baking pan, and fill it with the batter. Bake on the middle rack of the oven for 35 to 40 minutes, until a toothpick or knife blade inserted in the center comes out clean.

YIELD: Serves 12
SODIUM CONTENT: 15 mg. of sodium per serving

FRUIT SALAD WITH PORT

INGREDIENTS
- 2 peaches, peeled and sliced
- 1 small bunch seedless grapes, stems removed
- 2 bananas, sliced
- 1 pint fresh strawberries, halved
- 2 tbsp. port wine
- 1 tbsp. brandy (optional)

DIRECTIONS:
1. Place all the ingredients in a bowl and toss them together gently. Chill before serving.

YIELD: Serves 4
SODIUM CONTENT: 3 mg. of sodium per serving

PEARS IN WINE

- 4 Bosc pears
- 1 c. Chianti wine
- 1 c. sugar
- 2 tbsp. honey

DIRECTIONS:
1. Preheat the oven to 350 degrees. Place the pears upright in a baking dish and pour in the wine and sugar. Bake for 1 hour.
2. Remove the pears to a plate and cover lightly with aluminum foil. Allow the sauce to stand and cool; as it does, it will thicken up. Place a pear on a serving dish and spoon sauce over it, followed by about 1/2 tablespoon of honey.

YIELD: Serves 4
SODIUM CONTENT: 5 mg. of sodium per serving

POACHED PEACHES

- **Ingredients**
- 4 peaches
- 6 c. water
- 2 c. sugar
- 1/4 c. lemon juice

DIRECTIONS:
1. Place all the ingredients in a saucepan, and bring to a boil. Reduce the heat to a simmer and cook, covered, for 1 hour.
2. Remove the peaches from the pot; turn up the heat to medium and cook the liquid until it reduces to a syrup. Allow it to cool slightly. Peel each peach and slice it into wedges. To serve, arrange the wedges on 4 plates, and pour syrup over them.

YIELD: Serves 4
SODIUM CONTENT: 1 mg. of sodium per serving

DRUNKEN BANANAS

- **Ingredients**
- 2 bananas
- juice of 1 lemon
- 1/2 c. brown sugar
- 1/2 c. dark rum
- 1/4 tsp. cinnamon

DIRECTIONS:
1. Cut the bananas in half, then divide each half lengthwise. Place the lemon juice, sugar, rum, and cinnamon in a sauté pan and cook over medium heat until reduced to a syrup. Drop the pieces of banana in the pan and cook them for a few minutes in the syrup, turning them so they are completely coated. To serve, place two pieces of banana on a plate and spoon some of the syrup over them.

YIELD: Serves 4
SODIUM CONTENT: 9 mg. of sodium per serving

MAPLE WALNUT BAKED APPLES

- **Ingredients**
- 1/2 c. raisins and hot water to cover
- 4 large apples

- 1/2 c. chopped walnuts
- 1/2 c. maple syrup
- 1 tbsp. lemon juice
- 2 tbsp. unsalted butter
- 1 c. apple juice or water

DIRECTIONS:
1. Put the raisins in a bowl; cover with hot water and allow to stand for an hour, or until soft.
2. Preheat the oven to 375 degrees. Core each apple, leaving about 1/2 inch of flesh at the base of the hole you create. Take care not to poke through the bottom of the apple. Beginning at the edge of the hole in the top of the apple, peel away the skin about a third of the way down.
3. Drain the raisins, then put them in a small bowl with the walnuts, and stir to combine. Set the apples in a shallow baking pan and pack each core loosely with the walnut mixture, then pour in maple syrup to fill. Sprinkle a little lemon juice over each apple, then drizzle a bit more maple syrup on the exposed flesh. Place a thin slice of butter on the packed core of each apple. Pour the apple juice or water into the pan so it covers the bottom to a shallow depth. Bake on the middle rack of the oven until the apples are cooked through (test with a toothpick); this should take 35 to 40 minutes.

YIELD : Serves 4
SODIUM CONTENT: 11 mg. of sodium per serving

LIGHT LEMON SAUCE

INGREDIENTS
- 1/2 c. sugar
- 1 tbsp. cornstarch
- 1 c. water
- 1/4 c. lemon juice
- 2 tsp. grated lemon rind

DIRECTIONS:
1. Stir the sugar and cornstarch together in a saucepan until well blended. Add the water, lemon juice, and lemon rind, and stir to combine. Bring the mixture to a boil, continuing to stir until it thickens. Serve warm.

YIELD : Serves 4
SODIUM CONTENT: less than 1 mg. of sodium per serving

UNFORGETTABLE FUDGE SAUCE

INGREDIENTS
- 3 to 4 oz. high-quality bittersweet chocolate

- 12-oz. can evaporated skimmed milk
- 1/2 c. sugar
- 1 tsp. vanilla
- 2 tsp. cinnamon
- 2 tbsp. brewed coffee

DIRECTIONS:

1. Directionn a medium saucepan, melt the chocolate in the evaporated milk over moderate heat, stirring constantly. When all of the chocolate has melted, stir in the sugar, vanilla, and cinnamon. Continue to cook just under the boil, stirring frequently, until the sauce begins to thicken. Add the brewed coffee, and return the sauce to the heat, continuing to stir. When bubbles rise and burst slowly, as if in a lava flow, the sauce is thick enough to serve.

YIELD : Serves 6
SODIUM CONTENT: 70 mg. of sodium per serving

GOOD MACAROONS

INGREDIENTS

- 2 egg whites
- 1/2 c. sugar
- 3 tbsp. honey
- 1 tsp. vanilla extract
- 1 tsp. almond extract
- 1/3 c. flour
- 3 c. unsweetened dried coconut

DIRECTIONS:

1. Preheat the oven to 375 degrees. Beat the egg whites until they are soft, then stir in the sugar, honey, and vanilla and almond extract. Use a mixer to beat the mixture until it is very stiff. (This will take at least 10 minutes.) Fold in the flour and coconut and stir to distribute them evenly. Drop spoonfuls of the mixture onto a greased baking sheet. Bake on the top shelf of the oven for about 10 minutes or until the macaroons turn golden brown. Allow them to cool before removing them to a rack

2. These are excellent when coated with semisweet chocolate. Melt the chocolate in a pan, and dip each macaroon into it so it is half covered with the chocolate. Place on waxed paper until the chocolate has cooled and hardened. Serve with fresh strawberries.

YIELD : 12 macaroons
SODIUM CONTENT: 13 mg. of sodium per macaroon

CURRANT COCONUT CASHEW

COOKIES

INGREDIENTS

- 1/2 c. unsweetened dried coconut
- 1/2 c. (1 stick) unsalted butter
- 1/2 c. sugar
- 1 egg, lightly beaten
- 2 tbsp. honey
- 1 tsp. vanilla
- 1 1/4 c. all-purpose flour
- 1 tbsp. low-sodium baking powder
- 2/3 c. chopped cashews
- 1/2 c. dried currants

DIRECTIONS:

1. Preheat the oven to 350 degrees. Spread the coconut on a baking sheet and put it in the oven to toast for a few minutes until it begins to turn golden brown. Cream the butter and sugar together, then add the egg, honey, and vanilla, and stir to combine. Sift together the flour and baking powder in a large bowl. Add the toasted coconut, cashews, and currants, and stir to combine. Add the liquid ingredients, and stir to blend. Drop walnut-sized balls of batter onto a lightly greased baking sheet, and bake on the middle rack of the oven until the cookies begin to brown, about 15 minutes.

YIELD: 32 cookies
SODIUM CONTENT: 4 mg. of sodium per cookie

LEMON COCONUT COOKIES

INGREDIENTS

- 1/2 c. shredded unsweetened coconut
- 1/2 c. (1 stick) unsalted butter
- 1/2 c. sugar
- 1/4 c. maple syrup
- 1 egg
- zest of 1 lemon
- 3 tbsp. lemon juice
- 1 c. flour
- 1 tbsp. low-sodium baking powder

DIRECTIONS:

1. Preheat the oven to 350 degrees. Spread the coconut in a baking pan and toast in the oven until golden brown. Cream together the butter, sugar, and maple syrup. Add the egg, and stir to combine. Add the lemon zest and lemon juice. Stir in the toasted coconut. Sift together the flour and baking powder in a small bowl or on a sheet of waxed paper. Add to the liquid ingredients and stir to combine. Drop teaspoonfuls of the batter onto a lightly greased baking sheet. Cook on the middle rack of the oven until the edges of the cookies begin to turn brown and they resist on the top when touched with a fingertip.

YIELD: 24 cookies
  SODIUM CONTENT: 4 mg. of sodium per cookie

MOLASSES COOKIES

INGREDIENTS

- 1 c. sugar
- 3/4 c. unsalted butter or margarine
- 1/4 c. molasses
- 1 egg
- 2 c. flour
- 1 tbsp. low-sodium baking powder
- 1 tsp. cinnamon
- 3/4 tsp. ground ginger
- 3/4 tsp. ground cloves

DIRECTIONS:

1. Preheat the oven to 375 degrees. Cream the sugar with the butter or margarine, then stir in the molasses and egg. Sift together the flour, baking powder, and spices. Mix the dry ingredients with the wet, stirring to combine them well. Drop balls of dough the size of walnuts onto a lightly greased baking sheet. Bake on the middle rack of the oven for 10 to 12 minutes, until the tops are no longer puffed up and soft.

YIELD: 16 cookies
  SODIUM CONTENT: 10 mg. of sodium per cookie

OUR FAVORITE OATMEAL COOKIE

INGREDIENTS

- 1 1/2 c. all-purpose flour
- 1 tbsp. low-sodium baking powder
- 1 tsp. cinnamon
- 1 c. (2 sticks) melted unsalted butter or vegetable shortening
- 1 tbsp. molasses

- 1 c. sugar
- 1 egg
- 1/4 c. milk
- 13/4 c. uncooked rolled oats
- 1/2 c. raisins

DIRECTIONS:

1. Preheat the oven to 350 degrees. Sift the flour, baking powder, and cinnamon together in a mixing bowl. Combine the melted butter or shortening with the molasses and sugar in a small bowl, then stir into the flour mixture. Whisk the egg together with the milk, and stir into the batter. Fold in the rolled oats and raisins. Drop teaspoonsful of the batter onto a lightly greased cookie sheet, and bake for 10 to 15 minutes. When the edges turn brown, remove from the oven and place on a rack to cool.

YIELD: 18 cookies
SODIUM CONTENT: 9 mg. of sodium per cookie

PEANUT BUTTER COOKIES

INGREDIENTS

- 1/2 c. brown sugar
- 1/2 c. white sugar
- 1/2 c. (1 stick) unsalted butter, softened
- 1 egg
- 1 tsp. vanilla
- 1 c. salt-free peanut butter
- 2 tsp. low-sodium baking powder
- 11/4 c. all-purpose flour

DIRECTIONS:

1. Preheat the oven to 350 degrees. Cream together the sugars and butter until thoroughly blended. Stir in the egg and vanilla, followed by the peanut butter. Sift together the baking powder and flour; add to the wet ingredients, and stir to blend. To make the classic cookie, roll the dough into balls, drop them on a greased baking sheet, and press them flat with a fork to create a crosshatch pattern. If you wish, you may also roll out this dough to a thickness of 1/4 inch and use a glass to cut circles or cookie cutters to cut shapes.

YIELD: 12 cookies
SODIUM CONTENT: 12 mg. of sodium per cookie

AUNT LEN'S CHRISTMAS COOKIES

INGREDIENTS

- 1/2 c. (1 stick) unsalted butter
- 1/2 c. brown sugar
- 1 egg
- 1/2 c. light molasses
- 1 tbsp. crushed anise seeds
- 1 tsp. cinnamon
- 1 tsp. nutmeg
- 1 tsp. ground cloves
- 1/4 c. bourbon whiskey
- 1 c. finely chopped dates
- 1 c. golden raisins
- 1 c. roughly chopped walnuts
- 2 1/2 to 3 c. all-purpose flour
- 2 tsp. low-sodium baking powder

DIRECTIONS:

1. Cream together the butter and brown sugar. Stir in the egg and molasses. Add the anise seeds, cinnamon, nutmeg, and cloves, and stir to blend. Stir in the bourbon, followed by the dates, raisins, and walnuts. Sift the flour with the baking powder, and stir into the moist ingredients. Put the dough in the refrigerator to chill for 15 minutes.
2. Preheat the oven to 350 degrees. Use a rolling pin to roll out the dough on a floured board to a thickness of 1/4 inch in the shape of a large rectangle. (You may want to divide the dough into pieces and roll out each piece.) Cut individual cookies into rectangular shapes measuring about 2 inches by 3 inches. Place the cookies on a lightly greased baking sheet, and bake for 10 to 15 minutes, until they are cooked through and the edges turn slightly brown.

YIELD: 18 cookies
SODIUM CONTENT: 11 mg. of sodium per cookie

PECAN PUFFS

Ingredients

- 1/2 c. (1 stick) unsalted butter
- 2 tbsp. sugar
- 1 tsp. vanilla
- 1 c. finely ground pecans
- 1 c. plus 2 tbsp. all-purpose flour
- confectioners' sugar

DIRECTIONS:

1. Preheat the oven to 300 degrees. Cream the butter with the sugar. Add the vanilla and ground pecans, and stir to blend. Add the flour, and stir until evenly incorporated. Shape small pieces of the dough into balls about 1 inch in diameter. Place them on a lightly greased cookie sheet. Bake until slightly brown, about 30 to 40 minutes. While still warm, roll each puff in confectioners' sugar so that it is completely coated. Allow to cool completely, then dust each puff with confectioners' sugar a second time, covering areas where the first coating of sugar melted.

YIELD : 12 puffs
SODIUM CONTENT: 1 mg. of sodium per puff

THE BEST BROWNIES

INGREDIENTS

- 2 eggs
- 3/4 c. sugar
- 1 tsp. vanilla
- 1/2 c. (1 stick) unsalted butter, melted
- 2/3 c. sifted flour
- 3/4 c. ground sweet chocolate
- 1 tsp. low-sodium baking powder
- 1/2 c. semisweet chocolate chips or coarsely chopped bittersweet chocolate
- 1/2 c. coarsely chopped walnuts (optional)

DIRECTIONS:

1. Preheat oven to 350 degrees. Stir together the eggs, sugar, and vanilla in a large bowl. Add the melted butter. Sift the flour, ground chocolate, and baking powder together onto a piece of waxed paper. Stir these dry ingredients into the egg mixture; add chocolate chips or pieces and walnuts, and stir to distribute. Spread the mixture in a greased 9" × 9" baking pan and bake for 20 to 30 minutes, until you can stick a toothpick or knife blade into the center of the batter and it comes out clean. Allow to cool before cutting into brownies.

YIELD : 12 brownies
SODIUM CONTENT: 16 mg. of sodium per brownie

SNICKERDOODLES

- **INGREDIENTS**
- 1 c. sugar
- 1/2 c. (1 stick) butter or shortening
- 1 egg
- 1/2 tsp. vanilla

- 1 tbsp. low-sodium baking powder
- 1/2 c. milk
- 12-oz. package semisweet chocolate bits
- 2 c. sifted all-purpose flour
- 2 tbsp. cinnamon
- 2 tbsp. sugar

DIRECTIONS:

1. Preheat the oven to 350 degrees. Cream the sugar with the shortening or butter, stir in the egg and vanilla. Stir the baking powder into the milk and add it to the shortening-sugar mixture, stirring to blend thoroughly. Add the chocolate bits and stir to distribute, then add the flour, stirring until well blended. Spread the mixture in a lightly greased 9" × 12" baking tin, and sprinkle cinnamon and sugar over the top. Bake for about 30 minutes, until a toothpick or knife blade inserted into the center of the batter comes out clean. Allow to cool and then cut into bars.

YIELD: 12 bars
SODIUM CONTENT: 17 mg. of sodium per bar

Printed in Great Britain
by Amazon